50+ Quick & Easy, Instant Pot, Vegan, Vegetarian & Whole Food Plant-Based Recipes

by

GEOFF & VICKY WELLS

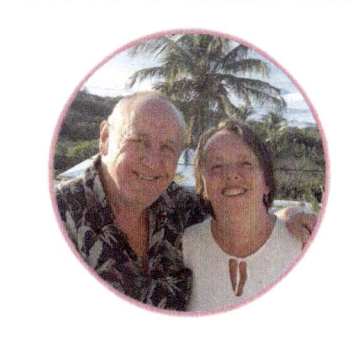

LIVING LIFE ON THE VEG

Copyright© 2020 by Geoff & Vicky Wells

All rights reserved

No part of this book may be used or reproduced in any manner whatsoever without prior written permission from the publisher, except for the inclusion of brief quotations in reviews.

Cover Artwork & Design by

Old Geezer Designs

Published in the United States by Reluctant Vegetarians

an imprint of DataIsland Software LLC,

Grand Portage, Minnesota
ISBN: 9798572307641

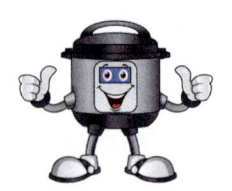

https://geezerguides.com

All product and company names are trademarks™ or registered® trademarks of their respective holders. Use of them does not imply any affiliation with or endorsement by them.

Table of Contents

Introduction 1

Breakfast Recipes

Fruity Oatmeal 9
Tutti Frutti Oatmeal (Using the Pot-in-Pot Method) 12
Cinnamon Quinoa 15

Main Dish Recipes

Africa-Inspired Peanut Vegetable Stew 19
Hearty Barley and Lentil Stew 23
Black Beans & Rice 26
Cauliflower Broccoli Stew 28
Jackfruit Curry Stew 31
Lentil Chili 34
Vicky's Instant Pot Red Beans and Rice 37
Kitchen Sink Cabbage Stew 39
Red Lentil & Greens Curry 41
Instant Pot Italian Bean Casserole 43
Spicy Lentils with Potato and Spinach 45
Eggplant and Sweet Potato Curry 47
Lentil Stuffed Peppers 50
Detox Cabbage Stew 54
Sicilian-Style Fava Beans 59
Cremini Pot Roast 63

Side Dish Recipes

Red Cabbage and Apple 68
Cauliflower Tikka Masala 71
Brown Rice Risotto with Sugar Snap Peas 74
Easy, Pot-In-Pot, Brown Rice 77

Soup Recipes

Asian Style Corn Soup 81
Creamy Tomato Soup 83
Detox Vegetable and Red Lentil Soup 86
Lentil and Yam Soup 89

Italian Inspired Pasta Soup 92
Black Bean Soup 95
Quick Potato Corn Chowder 97
French Onion Soup 99
White Bean & Beet Greens Soup 103
Creamy Potato Leek Soup 106
Split Pea and Potato Soup 108
Mung Bean Soup 111
Lima Bean Soup 113
Minestrone Soup 115
Instant Pot Mulligatawny Soup 119
Simple Cabbage Soup 122
Garlic Soup 124

Sauce Recipes

Red Lentil Mushroom Ragu 127
Fresh Tomato Marinara Sauce 130
Fresh Tomato Basil Sauce 133

Dessert Recipes

Rice Pudding 137
Easy Cheesecake for 2 (or 4) 139
Lemon Curd 143
Cinnamon Apples Using the Pot-in-Pot Method 146

Misc Recipes

Seasoned Diced Tomatoes 150
Corn Salsa 153
Easy Refried Beans 156
No Soak Beans 159
Homemade Vegetable Broth 162

Bonus Section

Just One More Thing 166
Other Books In The Reluctant Vegetarian Series 167

INTRODUCTION

More and more of us are using the Instant Pot to make deliciously easy meals that help us to get healthy, lose weight and save the planet.

We have certainly embraced this popular kitchen appliance phenomenon! We are the proud owners of FOUR - at last count!

Given that we are totally hooked on this way of cooking, we thought we'd like to share some of our favorite recipes to date. We continue to experiment and don't plan on stopping any time soon.

Vicky, who has yet to meet a kitchen appliance she doesn't like, has even insisted on taking at least one Instant Pot with us on vacation. No, I'm not kidding! It's usually the 6-quart Duo that tags along. So far, the 6-quart has been to Toronto, the Bahamas and British Columbia. I think she would have taken it to Europe, too, except that our version won't work there because Europe is 220V and our Instant Pot wants 110V.

Instant Pot terms - NPR, QR, etc.

The Instant Pot has some frequently used short forms and it's best to know what they mean when you're reading recipes.

QR - stands for **Quick Release** - what this means is, once the cooking time is complete, you want to release the pressure quickly. You do this by CAREFULLY moving the Pressure Valve from Sealing to Venting to release the pressure immediately.

Be aware that a lot of steam is going to be released through the Pressure Valve, so be prepared for that.

When we do a Quick Release we like to make sure our Instant Pot is turned so that the steam will be released into the center of the room and not under the cabinets.

Instant Pot recommends that you DO NOT cover the Pressure Valve. We've seen lots of recipes that tell you to cover the Pressure Valve with a towel - not a good idea.

TIP: Sometimes, when you do a Quick Release, some of the contents of the pot will begin to spew out of the Pressure Valve at the same time. If this happens, just turn the valve back to Sealing and give the contents a couple more minutes to settle down, then turn the valve back to Venting and you should be fine. Alternately, you can release some of the pressure in short bursts by lightly pressing down on the Pressure Valve a few times.

WARNING: - We have seen many examples on social media of people venting their Instant Pot by placing it on their stove and venting into the range hood. Sometimes the burners are still hot and other times people forget and leave the Instant Pot sitting on the stove. They knock the dial which turns on the burner underneath the IP. It's amazing how many times this happens. You wouldn't put your vacuum cleaner on the stove so why would you do that to your Instant Pot?

NPR - stands for **Natural Pressure Release** - what this means is once the cooking time is complete, you just let your Instant Pot sit until the Float Valve drops on its own. This is also sometimes referred to as Full NPR.

There's also a **Timed NPR** - what this means is that you let your Instant Pot sit for a specified amount of time after the cooking time is complete. For example, a 10-minute NPR means that you let your Instant Pot sit for 10 minutes once the cooking time is complete and then release the rest of the pressure using a QR (Quick Release).

PIP – stands for Pot in Pot

See Tutti Frutti Oatmeal pics for some pics of pot-in-pot

Using the Pot-in-Pot method means you put the items you are cooking in a separate bowl that sits on a trivet in the inner liner of your Instant Pot.

Be sure to put the correct amount of water in the inner pot before placing the trivet and bowl in the liner – 1 cup for a 6-quart Instant Pot and 2 cups for an 8-quart Instant Pot. You need the water to build the pressure.

Note: If you don't want water from the steam to get onto whatever you are cooking, then cover the dish with a lid of some sort. We have several silicone lids for just this purpose.

How to Make a Foil Sling for Your Instant Pot

When using the Pot-in-Pot method, there will be times when the bowl/container you use will be a bit of a snug fit. Just, make sure it's not TOO snug.

There always needs to be some space between the container you are using and the walls of the inner liner.

The steam needs to be able to circulate properly for your Instant Pot to be able to come up to pressure.

However, that may mean that there just isn't enough room to place the container on the trivet using your fingers.

That's where a sling comes in.

Now, there are some silicone slings that can be purchased for your Instant Pot, but we find that making a foil sling is easy and a lot less expensive.

Here's how to make one:

Use a length of aluminum foil that is long enough to go around the bottom of the container you are using and have the ends come up over the top once the container is placed on the trivet. So, about 12 - 18 inches (30 - 45 cm) long.

Lay it flat on your counter and then fold the long ends so each edge meets in the center. Then fold in half lengthwise. This way you have a long strip of foil that is four layers thick.

You can use this to carefully place it under the container you are using and gently lower it onto the trivet and just leave it in your Instant Pot. Fold the ends over the container, if necessary, to close the lid of the Instant Pot.

When the cooking time is done and you have removed the lid of the Instant Pot, use the foil sling to carefully remove the container from the trivet.

Vegetables in the Instant Pot

We tend to steam our vegetables mostly, rather than do them in the Instant Pot.

Why? Well, it's very easy to overcook vegetables in an Instant Pot.

We've been horrified at some recipe books we've seen that give instructions that would result in your veggies being, basically, mush! One recipe we noticed recently, said to cook cubed potatoes for 10 minutes on Pressure Cook/Manual followed by a FULL NPR! Nope - that's a recipe for mush.

We've had a lot of hit-and-miss trials trying to cook vegetables in our Instant Pot. We like our veggies tender-crisp and that's really hard to achieve in an Instant Pot.

Don't forget, while your pot is coming up to pressure, those vegetables have already started to cook.

That's why we mostly use a steamer to cook our veggies - so we can check them during the cooking process.

Rice in the Instant Pot

Since getting our Instant Pot, we don't cook rice any other way. It, quite simply, comes out perfect every time.

Our favorite way to cook it is using the pot-in-pot method. For an explanation of how that's done, check out our Easy, Pot-In-Pot, Brown Rice recipe below.

Yes, there's a Rice button on the Instant Pot. That's only used for white rice (check your manual), and we don't normally cook white rice. We prefer to have whole-grain brown rice.

If you do want to cook white rice using the Rice function, just follow the instructions in your Instant Pot manual.

Which Instant Pot We Used

Unless otherwise noted, these recipes were made in a 6-quart Instant Pot Duo.

The Pressure Cook/Manual Button

In many of the recipes, you'll be instructed to use the Pressure Cook/Manual button. However, the button will be labeled with EITHER Pressure Cook or Manual, not both.

Older Instant Pots will have the Manual button. Newer Instant Pots will have the Pressure Cook button.

We found that some people who had newer Instant Pots were getting confused by recipes that instructed them to use the Manual button.

If you see some of these older recipes, the Pressure Cook button is the same thing as the Manual button.

The Instant Pot Can't Do Everything

While the Instant Pot is an amazing kitchen appliance (pretty much our favorite) that does a lot of things very, very well, that doesn't mean that it can do EVERYTHING well.

Always use the right tool for the job.

Budget Friendly

There seems to be a misconception that switching to a vegan, vegetarian or WFPB diet is expensive. This just isn't true.

Remember, you're eliminating meat (and generally dairy, too) from your grocery shopping and meat can be very expensive.

Now, if you opt to purchase a lot of processed vegan foods, well, yes, that can get VERY expensive.

It's best to stick to Whole Foods Plant-Based (that's right – WFPB) and avoid anything pre-packaged.

You'll get the best bang for your buck that way as well as fresh, healthy, whole foods.

This is How We Eat

We have made each and every recipe in this book and this is how we actually eat on a day-to-day basis.

No, not all of our meals are prepared in an Instant Pot, but a good portion of them are.

ABOUT THE RECIPES

Vegan/Vegetarian/WFPB

Each recipe will be designated with at least one of these terms. And here's what they all mean:

Vegan: If a recipe is designated as Vegan, it will also be suitable for Vegetarians but it may or may not be WFPB. The reason some Vegan recipes may not be WFPB is that there are a lot of Vegan foods that are highly processed and, therefore, cannot be considered a "whole food." That includes things like refined sugar (yes, that's vegan), processed oils from plant sources (coconut oil, olive oil, etc.) and prepackaged vegan items like veggie sausages, burgers, etc.

Vegetarian: If a recipe is designated as Vegetarian that means it includes something that is NOT considered Vegan, such as dairy products.

WFPB: This acronym stands for Whole Food Plant-Based. Given this designation, you can be pretty sure that anything WFPB will also be Vegan. All this actually means is that any recipe designated WFPB includes only items that stay as close to the actual whole food as possible.

Note: You may also see it designated as WFPBNO (Whole Food Plant-Based No Oil).

Oil-Free

Wherever possible, we have endeavored to make the recipes oil-free. After much experimentation, we have found that omitting the oil in most of the recipes resulted in no difference in taste but reduced the calories. Sometimes, in the past, we have just added oil/butter to recipes as a matter of habit without thinking whether or not it was really necessary. We are happy to report that, in most of the recipes, nothing is added or lost by removing the oil/butter.

Nutritional Information

We use a program called MacGourmet to record all of our recipes. This program includes a nutritional database, which is tied into the USDA nutritional database, and that's what we use for all the nutritional information including the calorie counts.

Each recipe shows a long list of nutrients. This may seem like a bit of overkill but we've had many people ask us for nutritional information on our recipes and rather than pick and choose which nutrients to show, we've included everything.

Total Cooking Times

When using an Instant Pot, the "cook" time can sometimes be misleading. Lots of recipes proclaim - "Cooks in only 4 minutes!" - but this is only part of the story.

With your Instant Pot there are other factors to consider that add to the overall time it takes to result in a completed dish.

You have to consider the time it takes to come to pressure, the length of the NPR (Natural Pressure Release) once the cooking time is complete and then the time for the pressure to release whether you are using a QR (Quick Release) or a full NPR.

So, time to come to pressure + cooking time + time for pressure to release (whether NPR, QR or a timed NPR + QR) = total Instant Pot cooking time.

When we first started developing recipes for our Instant Pot, we didn't even think to make note of anything but the button to push, the cooking time and whether it was a Natural Pressure Release or a Quick Release.

So, a lot of the recipes do not have the COMPLETE cooking time.

However, once we realized that this was valuable information, we started to record these details. You'll find that some of the recipes will have a section called "Useful Information on total cooking time" that details the complete cooking time to make it easier to determine when your dish will be ready.

BREAKFAST RECIPES

FRUITY OATMEAL

| Vegan | Oil-free | WFPB | | Servings: 4 |

Oatmeal is often our go-to breakfast. This recipe is particularly tasty and easy to make, too.

INGREDIENTS

1 medium apple, chopped

½ teaspoon (2.5 ml) cinnamon

6 dates, pitted and chopped

2 tablespoons (30 ml) walnut pieces

2 tablespoons (30 ml) raisins

1 cup (80g) old fashion oatmeal

2¼ cups (535 ml) water

½ teaspoon (2.5 ml) vanilla

¼ teaspoon (1.25 ml) salt

DIRECTIONS

1. Add all of the ingredients to the inner pot of the Instant Pot and stir.
2. Close and lock the lid ensuring that the Pressure Valve is turned to the Sealing position.
3. Select Pressure Cook/Manual mode and set the cooking time for 4 minutes.
4. When cooking time is complete, allow a 10-minute NPR and then carefully turn the Pressure Valve to Venting.
5. When all the pressure has been released, and the Float Valve has dropped, carefully remove the lid.

6. Remove the inner pot to a heatproof surface.
7. Give the oatmeal a good stir and serve immediately.

Useful Information on total cooking time:

Time to come to pressure: approx. 6 minutes

Cooking time: 4 minutes

NPR: 10 minutes

QR: time for pressure to release: less than a minute

Total Instant Pot time: approx. 20 minutes

Nutritional Information Per Serving:

Nutritional Information per Serving	
Servings 4	
Calories: 259	**Total fat:** 4.71g
Calories from fat: 42 (16%)	Saturated: 0.72g
Total Carbohydrates: 48.42g	Monounsaturated: 1.19g
Dietary Fiber: 7.28g	Polyunsaturated: 2.80g
Sugars: 17.34g	Trans fat: NA
Cholesterol: --	**Sodium:** 152mg
Protein 7.76g	**Potassium** 368mg
Vitamin A: 42IU	**Vitamin C:** 3.63mg	**Calcium:** 40mg
Iron: 2.25mg	**Thiamin:** 0.33mg	**Niacin:** 0.66mg
Vitamin B6: 0.12mg	**Magnesium:** 85mg	**Folate:** 29µg

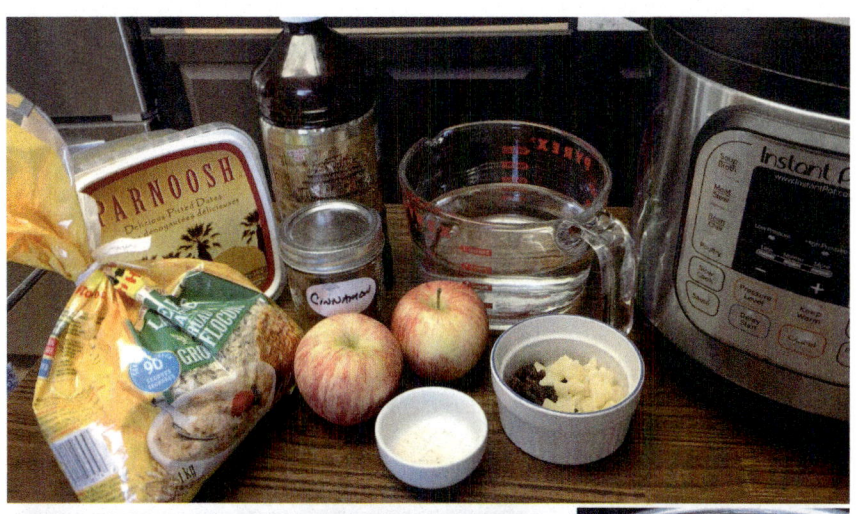

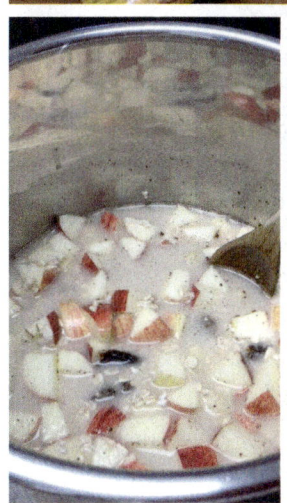

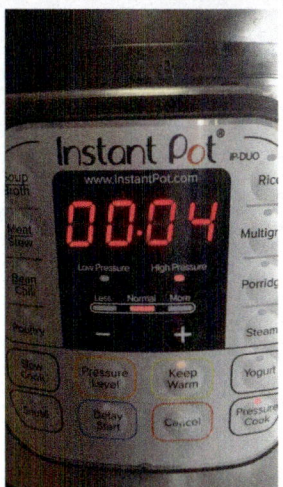

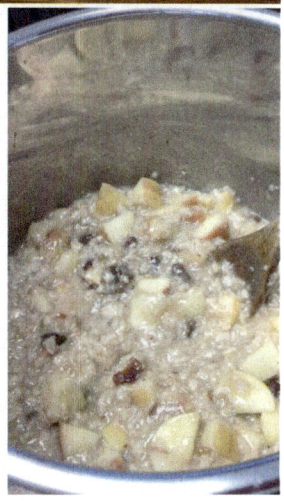

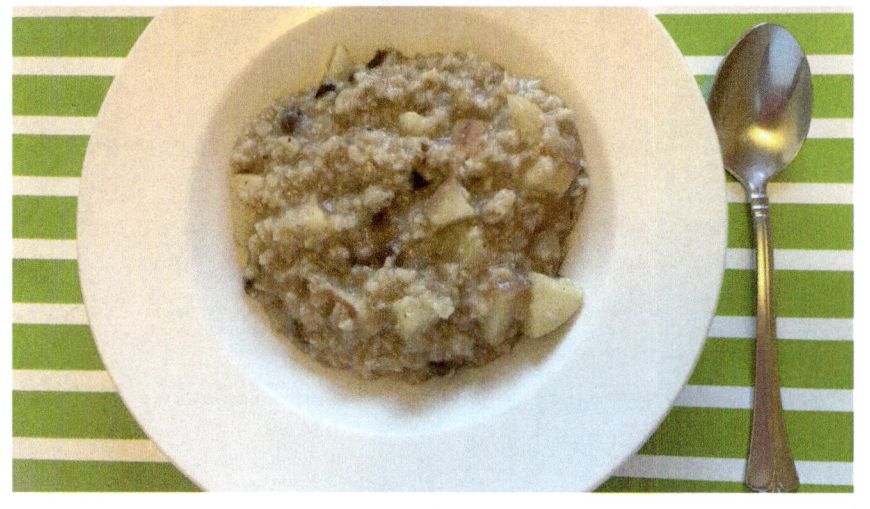

Tutti Frutti Oatmeal
(Using the Pot-in-Pot Method)

Vegan	Oil-free	WFPB		Servings: 4

We find that cooking oatmeal using the Pot-in-Pot method makes for easier clean up.

INGREDIENTS

2¼ cups (535 ml) water

1 cup (80g) old fashion oatmeal

¼ teaspoon (1.25 ml) cinnamon

6 dates, pitted and chopped

⅛ cup (20g) raisins

⅛ cup (15g) dehydrated pineapple chunks

⅛ cup (15g) dehydrated apple chunks

½ teaspoon (2.5 ml) vanilla

¼ teaspoon (1.25 ml) salt

DIRECTIONS

1. Add all of the ingredients to a bowl that will easily fit in your Instant Pot. Stir well.
2. Add 1 cup (240 ml) water and the trivet to the inner pot of your Instant Pot
3. Place the bowl on the trivet. Use a foil sling, if required. (See How to Make a Foil Sling for your Instant Pot)
4. Close and lock the lid ensuring that the Pressure Valve is turned to the Sealing position.

5. Select Pressure Cook/Manual mode and set the cooking time for 4 minutes.
6. When cooking time is complete, carefully turn the Pressure Valve to Venting.
7. When all the pressure has been released, and the Float Valve has dropped, carefully remove the lid.
8. Remove the inner pot to a heatproof surface and carefully remove the bowl using the foil sling.
9. Give the oatmeal a good stir and serve immediately.

Useful Information on Total Cooking Time:

Time to come to pressure: approx. 10 minutes

Cooking time: 4 minutes

QR: time for pressure to release: approx. 2 minutes

Total Instant Pot time: approx. 16 minutes

Nutritional Information per Serving:

Nutritional Information per Serving		
Servings 4		
Calories: 205	**Total fat:** 2.33g	
Calories from fat: 20 (10%)	Saturated: 0.48g	
Total Carbohydrates: 40.02g	Monounsaturated: 0.85g	
Dietary Fiber: 5.55g	Polyunsaturated: 0.99g	
Sugars: 9.50g	Trans fat: NA	
Cholesterol: --	**Sodium:** 154mg	
Protein 7.03g	**Potassium** 288mg	
Vitamin A: 3IU	**Vitamin C:** 0.23mg	**Calcium:** 32mg
Iron: 2.10mg	**Thiamin:** 0.31mg	**Niacin:** 0.57mg
Vitamin B6: 0.07mg	**Magnesium:** 76mg	**Folate:** 23µg

14

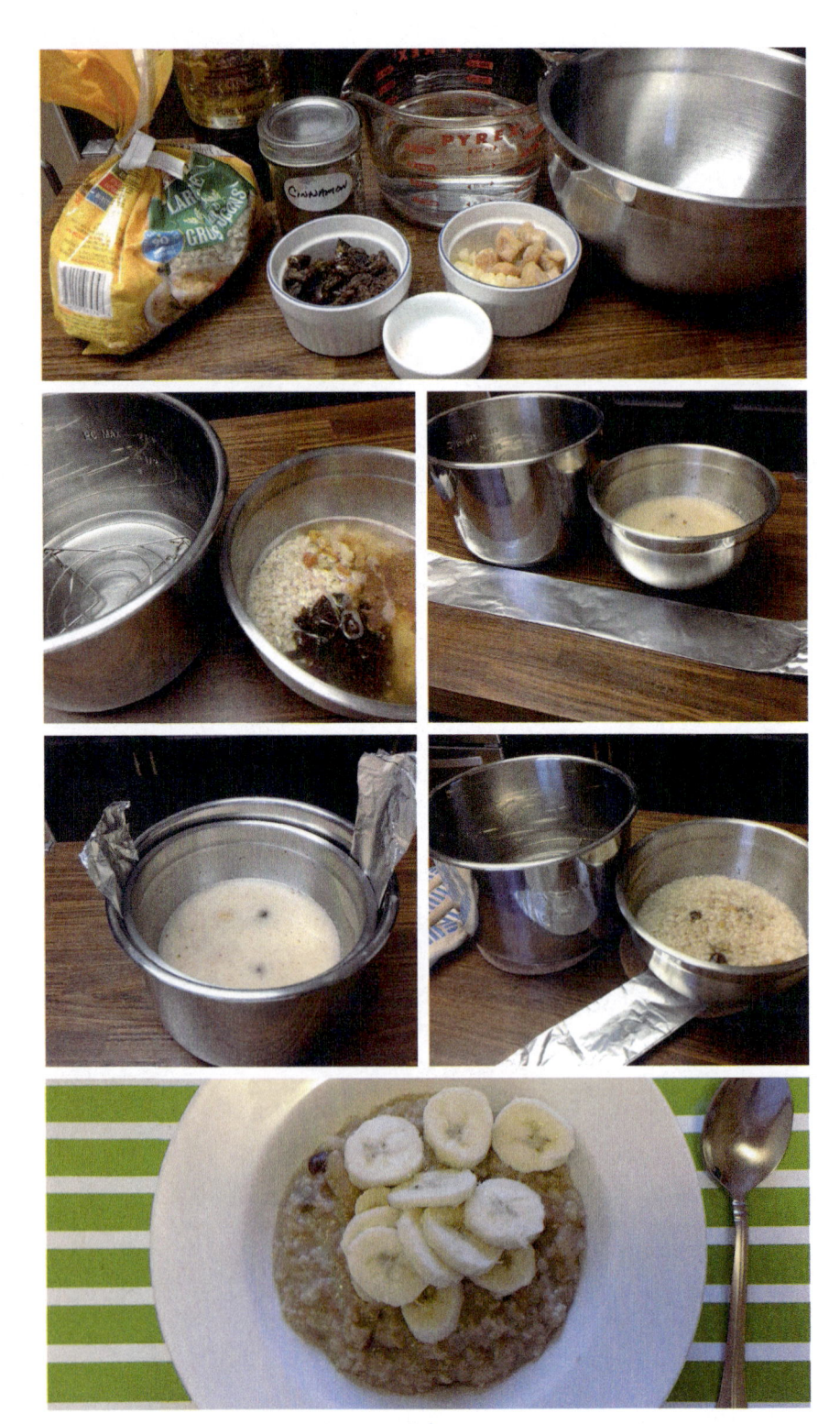

Cinnamon Quinoa

Vegan	Oil-free	WFPB		Servings: 4

A nice change from oatmeal, this recipe is creamy, tasty and nutritious. It cooks quickly (See the total time at the end of this recipe).

This recipe can be used for breakfast – served warm – or for dessert – served either warm or cold. It can also be easily doubled or even tripled.

Top the warm quinoa with chopped almonds, fresh fruit or unsweetened applesauce.

INGREDIENTS

½ cup (90g) quinoa, well-rinsed

½ cup (120 ml) almond milk

¾ cup (180 ml) water

½ teaspoon (2.5 ml) cinnamon

½ teaspoon (2.5 ml) vanilla extract

¼ cup (90g) dates, pitted and chopped

DIRECTIONS

1. Add all of the ingredients to the inner pot of the Instant Pot and stir.
2. Close and lock the lid ensuring that the Pressure Valve is turned to the Sealing position.
3. Select Pressure Cook/Manual mode and set the cooking time for 2 minutes.
4. Once the cooking time is complete, allow a 10-minute NPR (Natural Pressure Release). (That just means letting your Instant Pot

sit for 10 minutes.) Then release the rest of the pressure by carefully turning the Pressure Valve from Sealing to Venting.

5. When all the pressure has been released, and the Float Valve has dropped, carefully remove the lid.
6. Remove the inner pot to a heatproof surface.
7. Give the quinoa a good stir and serve immediately and add toppings if desired.

Useful Information on total cooking time:

Time to come to pressure: approx. 6 minutes

Cooking time: 2 minutes

NPR: 10 minutes

QR: time for pressure to release: less than a minute

Total Instant Pot time: approx. 18-19 minutes

Nutritional Information Per Serving:

Nutritional Information per Serving

Servings 4

Calories: 113

Calories from fat: 13 (12%)

Total Carbohydrates: 21.86g

  Dietary Fiber: 2.52g

  Sugars: 6.77g

Total fat: 1.51g

  Saturated: 0.15g

  Monounsaturated: 0.35g

  Polyunsaturated: 0.70g

  Trans fat: NA

Cholesterol: --

Protein 3.36g

Sodium: 21mg

Potassium 181mg

Vitamin A: 4IU	Vitamin C: 0.05mg	Calcium: 17mg
Iron: 1.09mg	Thiamin: 0.08mg	Niacin: 0.45mg
Vitamin B6: 0.12mg	Magnesium: 45mg	Folate: 40μg

17

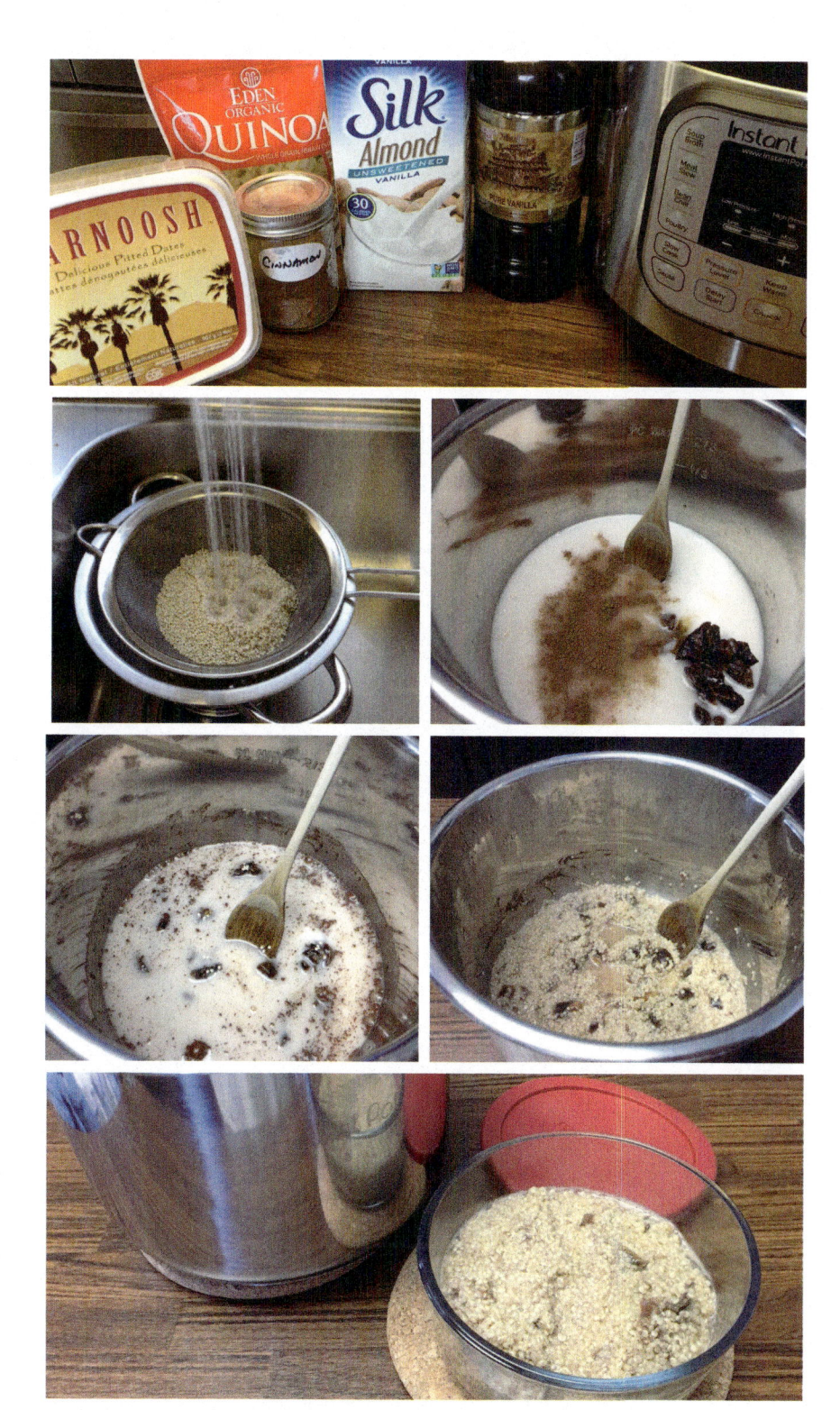

MAIN DISH RECIPES

AFRICA-INSPIRED PEANUT VEGETABLE STEW

Vegan	Oil-free	WFPB		Servings: 12

This hearty stew has an amazing flavor and fast became one of our favorite dishes. It provides as much, or as little, warmth as you like depending on how much (or how little) red pepper flakes and sriracha you choose to add. We like it to be medium warm so the "hot" doesn't overpower the actual taste.

We like to serve this stew over spaghetti but any pasta or rice will work well, too.

INGREDIENTS

1 large yellow onion, diced

3 medium carrots, chopped

1 large green bell pepper, chopped

16 ounces (454g) yams (sweet potatoes), peeled and chopped

5 cloves garlic, minced

1 teaspoon (5 ml) ginger, minced

¼ cup (60 ml) lime juice, preferably freshly squeezed

4 cups (950 ml) vegetable broth

½ cup (125g) natural peanut butter, smooth or chunky

3 cups (225g) navy beans, canned or home cooked, drained and rinsed

1 tablespoon (15 ml) dehydrated onion flakes

1 teaspoon (5 ml) garlic powder

1 teaspoon (5 ml) cumin

½ teaspoon (2.5 ml) red pepper flakes

28 ounces (828 ml) crushed tomatoes

2 tablespoons (30 ml) maple syrup

1 teaspoon (5 ml) salt

1 teaspoon (5 ml) pepper, freshly ground

1 teaspoon (5 ml) sriracha (optional), or to taste

4 cups (400g) baby spinach

GARNISH (OPTIONAL)

Peanuts, chopped and/or Spring onions, sliced

DIRECTIONS

1. Prepare all of the ingredients as listed.
2. Add all the ingredients to the inner liner of your Instant Pot with the exception of Maple Syrup, Salt, Pepper, Sriracha and Spinach. (They'll go in later.)
3. Make sure that the Crushed Tomatoes are the last thing you add to the pot and DO NOT STIR! That's because tomato products can result in a Burn Notice if they are in contact with the bottom of the pot.
4. Close and lock the lid ensuring that the Pressure Valve is in the Sealing position.
5. Select Soup/Broth mode and set the cooking time for 4 minutes.
6. Once cooking time is complete, allow a 10-minute NPR (Natural Pressure Release) to allow the contents to settle down a bit. Then carefully turn the Pressure Valve from Sealing to Venting to release the rest of the pressure.
7. When all of the pressure has been released, and the Float Valve has dropped, carefully remove the lid.
8. Carefully transfer the inner liner of your Instant Pot to a heatproof surface and give it a good stir.
9. Add the Maple Syrup, Salt, Pepper and Sriracha (if using) and stir well.
10. Add the baby spinach and stir until the spinach has wilted.
11. Serve over pasta or rice and garnish with the chopped peanuts and sliced spring onions, if desired.

Useful Information on total cooking time:

Time to come to pressure: approx. 31 minutes (Note: we used semi-frozen vegetable broth in this recipe.)

Cooking time: 4 minutes

NPR: 10 minutes

QR: time for pressure to release: approx. 4 minutes

Total Instant Pot time: 49 minutes

Nutritional Information Per Servings

Nutritional Information per Serving

Servings	12	
Calories: 218	**Total fat:** 5.25g	
Calories from fat: 47 (21%)	Saturated: 0.95g	
Total Carbohydrates: 35.79g	Monounsaturated: 2.56g	
Dietary Fiber: 8.13g	Polyunsaturated: 1.74g	
Sugars: 8.83g	Trans fat: NA	
Cholesterol: --	**Sodium:** 528mg	
Protein 8.90g	**Potassium** 943mg	
Vitamin A: 4318IU	**Vitamin C:** 37.52mg	**Calcium:** 92mg
Iron: 2.84mg	**Thiamin:** 0.20mg	**Niacin:** 3.21mg
Vitamin B6: 0.43mg	**Magnesium:** 75mg	**Folate:** 104μg

22

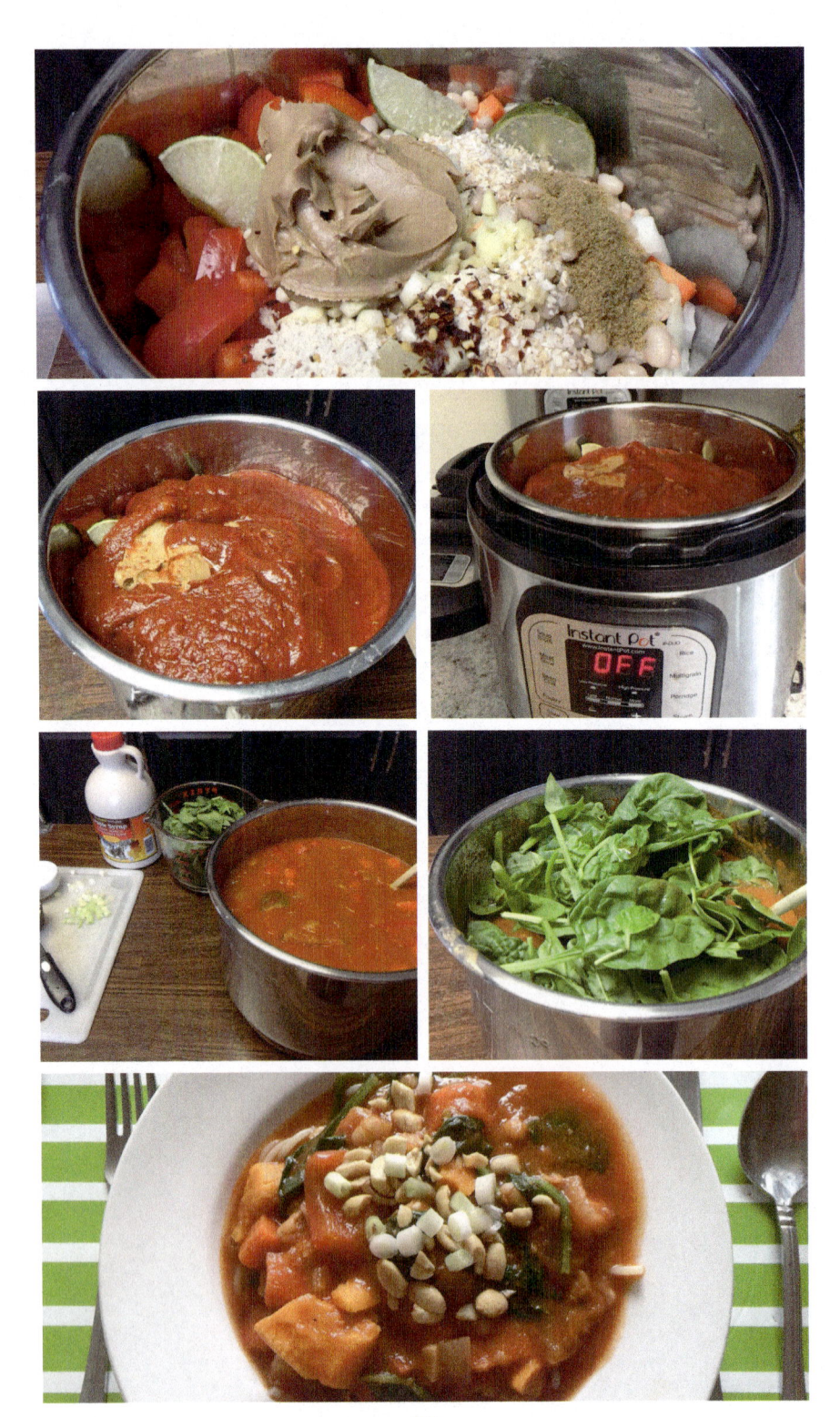

Hearty Barley and Lentil Stew

| Vegan | Oil-free | WFPB | | Servings: 8 |

Note: We used an 8-quart Instant Pot for this recipe.

This hearty vegan stew is also low calorie. It is a favorite comfort food of ours for a cool fall or winter day. Serve with some warm, freshly baked, crusty bread. Make your own vegetable broth if you can, the commercial types usually have too much salt and other ingredients you may not want. Just save all the peelings and cuttings and use your Instant Pot to make your own vegetable broth. We also save the water from any veggies we steam or boil.

INGREDIENTS

- 8 cups (1.9 L) vegetable broth
- 1 large yellow onion, coarsely chopped
- 2 large carrots, cut in chunks
- 1 large potato, cut in chunks, not peeled
- 2 ribs celery, sliced
- 2 cloves garlic, chopped
- ¾ cup (150g) pearl barley
- ¾ cup (150g) green lentils
- 4-6 leaves fresh basil, chopped
- 1 teaspoon (5 ml) fennel seeds
- 2 teaspoons (10 ml) black pepper, freshly ground
- 2 cups (200g) kale, chopped, or greens of your choice
- 1½ teaspoons (7.5 ml) sea salt

DIRECTIONS

1. Place all of the ingredients in your Instant Pot and stir well.
2. Select the Soup/Stew function and set the cooking time for 20 minutes.
3. Once cooking time is complete, allow a NPR (Natural Pressure Release) for 10-15 minutes. Then carefully release the rest of the pressure by turning the Pressure Valve from Sealing to Venting.
4. Once all of the pressure has been released and the Float Valve has dropped, carefully remove the lid.
5. Remove the inner liner to a heatproof surface and stir well.
6. Serve Immediately.
7. This dish goes well with some crusty bread.
8. Leftovers freeze well.

Useful Information on total cooking time:

Time to come to pressure: approx. 27 minutes (Note: we used semi-frozen vegetable broth in this recipe.)

Cooking time: 20 minutes

NPR: 15 minutes

QR: time for pressure to release: approx. 4 minutes

Total Instant Pot time: 1 hour 6 minutes

Nutritional Information per Serving:

Nutritional Information per Serving		
Servings 8		
Calories: 201	**Total fat:** 0.55g	
Calories from fat: 4 (2%)	Saturated: 0.12g	
Total Carbohydrates: 42.42g	Monounsaturated: 0.11g	
Dietary Fiber: 7.55g	Polyunsaturated: 0.32g	
Sugars: 4.87g	Trans fat: NA	
Cholesterol: --	**Sodium:** 1019mg	
Protein 8.42g	**Potassium** 566mg	
Vitamin A: 4653IU	**Vitamin C:** 20.18mg	**Calcium:** 68mg
Iron: 2.70mg	**Thiamin:** 0.26mg	**Niacin:** 2.24mg
Vitamin B6: 0.38mg	**Magnesium:** 51mg	**Folate:** 124µg

Black Beans & Rice

Vegan	Oil-free	WFPB		Servings: 8

Rice and beans dishes are a staple in our house. We love them!

INGREDIENTS

1 medium red onion, coarsely chopped

4 cloves of garlic, crushed and minced

1 tablespoon (15 ml) cumin

2 cups (450g) brown rice

2 cups (400g) dry black beans

1 jalapeño, seeded and chopped, optional

8 cups (1.9 L) vegetable broth or water

1 teaspoon (5 ml) salt (omit if you are using a commercial vegetable broth)

OPTIONAL GARNISH

Fresh lime juice

1 medium tomato chopped

¼ cup (40g) onion, chopped

¼ cup (15g) cilantro, chopped, optional (not everyone likes cilantro - Vicky loves it, Geoff hates it)

DIRECTIONS

1. Add all of the ingredients (with the exception of the garnish ingredients) to the inner liner of your Instant Pot.
2. Close and lock the lid ensuring the Pressure Valve is in the Sealing position.

3. Select the Multigrain function and set the cooking time to 22 minutes.
4. When cooking time is complete, allow a full Natural Pressure Release. That means letting the pressure come down on its own - it can take 30 minutes or more.
5. While waiting for the pressure to release, combine the chopped tomato, onion and cilantro in a small bowl and toss to mix.
6. Once all the pressure has been released and the Float Valve has dropped, carefully remove the lid and stir the rice and beans.
7. Serve in individual bowls, squeeze a little lime juice on each serving and top with a little of the tomato/onion/cilantro mixture.

Nutritional Information per Serving (includes garnish):

Nutritional Information per Serving		
Servings 8		
Calories: 362	**Total fat:** 1.65g	
Calories from fat: 14 (4%)	Saturated: 0.38g	
Total Carbohydrates: 73.43g	Monounsaturated: 0.61g	
Dietary Fiber: 9.56g	Polyunsaturated: 0.67g	
Sugars: 5.77g	Trans fat: NA	
Cholesterol: --	**Sodium** 1242mg	
Protein 14.11g	**Potassium** 936mg	
Vitamin A: 698IU	**Vitamin C:** 7.20mg	**Calcium:** 110mg
Iron: 5.56mg	**Thiamin:** 0.64mg	**Niacin:** 3.16mg
Vitamin B6: 0.47mg	**Magnesium:** 150mg	**Folate:** 226µg

Cauliflower Broccoli Stew

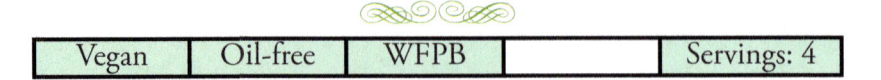

| Vegan | Oil-free | WFPB | | Servings: 4 |

This stew can be served with potatoes (baked, boiled, mashed), rice or pasta.

INGREDIENTS

1⅓ cups (320 ml) vegetable broth, preferably homemade

1 medium yellow onion, halved and sliced

3 cups (320g) cauliflower florets, bite-sized

2 cups (350g) broccoli florets, bite-sized

2 cups (125g) Romano beans, cooked, or your choice of cooked beans

1 medium jalapeño, seeded and chopped

1 tablespoon (15 ml) ginger, minced

1 tablespoon (15 ml) cumin

1 tablespoon (15 ml) garam masala

1 teaspoon (5 ml) turmeric

1 cup (100g) kale, chopped

2 cups (450g) diced tomatoes, canned with juice

2 cups (250g) mushrooms, halved or quartered, depending on size

½ cup (120 ml) coconut milk

2 teaspoons (10 ml) sea salt

2 tablespoons (30 ml) cilantro, chopped, optional

DIRECTIONS

1. Combine all the ingredients in the inner liner of your Instant Pot, with the exception of the coconut milk, salt and cilantro, and stir well.
2. Close and lock the lid ensuring the Pressure Valve is in the Sealing position.
3. Select Pressure Cook/Manual mode and set the cooking time for 2 minutes.
4. When cooking time is complete, allow a 2-minute NPR (Natural Pressure Release), then release the rest of the pressure by carefully turning the Pressure Valve from Sealing to Venting.
5. Once all the pressure has been released and the Float Valve has dropped, carefully remove the lid.
6. Add the coconut milk, salt and the optional cilantro. Stir well.
7. Thicken with a cornstarch slurry if necessary and serve immediately.
8. While you can freeze this dish, the vegetables will become pretty mushy when reheated.

Useful Information on total cooking time:

Time to come to pressure: approx. 23 minutes

Cooking time: 2 minutes

NPR: 2 minutes

QR: time for pressure to release: 2 minutes

Total Instant Pot time: approx. 29 minutes

Nutritional Information per Serving:

Nutritional Information per Serving			
Servings	4			
Calories: 323		Total fat: 7.60g		
Calories from fat: 68 (21%)		Saturated: 5.85g		
Total Carbohydrates: 51.75g		Monounsaturated: 0.91g		
Dietary Fiber: 13.94g		Polyunsaturated: 0.84g		
Sugars: 10.51g		Trans fat: NA		
Cholesterol: --	Sodium: 1946mg		
Protein: 17.11g	Potassium: 1410mg		
Vitamin A: 1982IU	Vitamin C: 95.32mg	Calcium: 206mg
Iron: 7.28mg	Thiamin: 0.28mg	Niacin: 4.29mg
Vitamin B6: 0.50mg	Magnesium: 123mg	Folate: 140µg

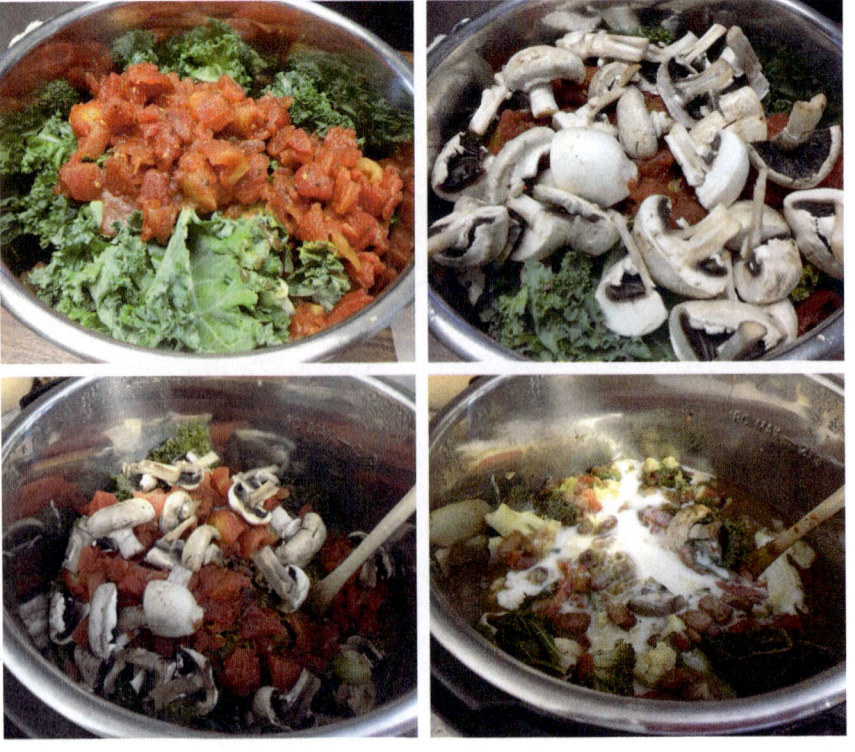

Jackfruit Curry Stew

| Vegan | Oil-free | WFPB | | Servings: 6 |

Jackfruit is fast becoming a popular vegan option. It lends itself to all kinds of dishes and adds texture while blending well with many different flavors.

INGREDIENTS

2 cups (475 ml) vegetable broth, preferably homemade

15 ounces (443 ml) coconut milk

2 tablespoons (30 ml) curry powder

1 teaspoon (5 ml) paprika

1 teaspoon (5 ml) cumin

1 teaspoon (5 ml) turmeric

1 cup (150g) onion, chopped

4 cloves garlic, minced

1 tablespoon (15 ml) ginger, grated

1 tablespoon (15 ml) Italian seasoning

¼ teaspoon (1.25 ml) cayenne pepper

1 medium carrot, diced

20 ounces (567g) jackfruit, canned, drained

DIRECTIONS

1. Add all of the ingredients to the inner liner of your Instant Pot. Stir well.
2. Close and lock the lid ensuring that the Pressure Valve is in the Sealing position.

3. Select Pressure Cook/Manual mode and set the cooking time for 10 minutes.
4. Once cooking time is complete, allow a 10 minute NPR (Natural Pressure Release) and then release the rest of the pressure by carefully turning the Pressure Valve from Sealing to Venting.
5. Once all of the pressure has been released, and the Float Valve has dropped, carefully remove the lid.
6. Stir well and serve immediately with your choice of side dishes.
7. Refrigerate or freeze any leftovers.

Useful Information on total cooking time:

Time to come to pressure: approx. 11 minutes

Cooking time: 10 minutes

NPR: 10 minutes

QR: time for pressure to release: approx. 3 minutes

Total Instant Pot time: approx. 34 minutes

Nutritional Information per Serving:

Nutritional Information per Serving

Servings	6		
Calories: 266		**Total fat:** 15.13g	
Calories from fat: 136 (51%)		Saturated: 13.69g	
Total Carbohydrates: 32.24g		Monounsaturated: 1.04g	
Dietary Fiber: 4.12g		Polyunsaturated: 0.40g	
Sugars: 20.52g		Trans fat: NA	
Cholesterol: --	**Sodium:** 204mg		
Protein 4.20g	**Potassium** 732mg		
Vitamin A: 2209IU	**Vitamin C:** 16.98mg	**Calcium:** 79mg	
Iron: 4.17mg	**Thiamin:** 0.14mg	**Niacin:** 1.72mg	
Vitamin B6: 0.42mg	**Magnesium:** 76mg	**Folate:** 42µg	

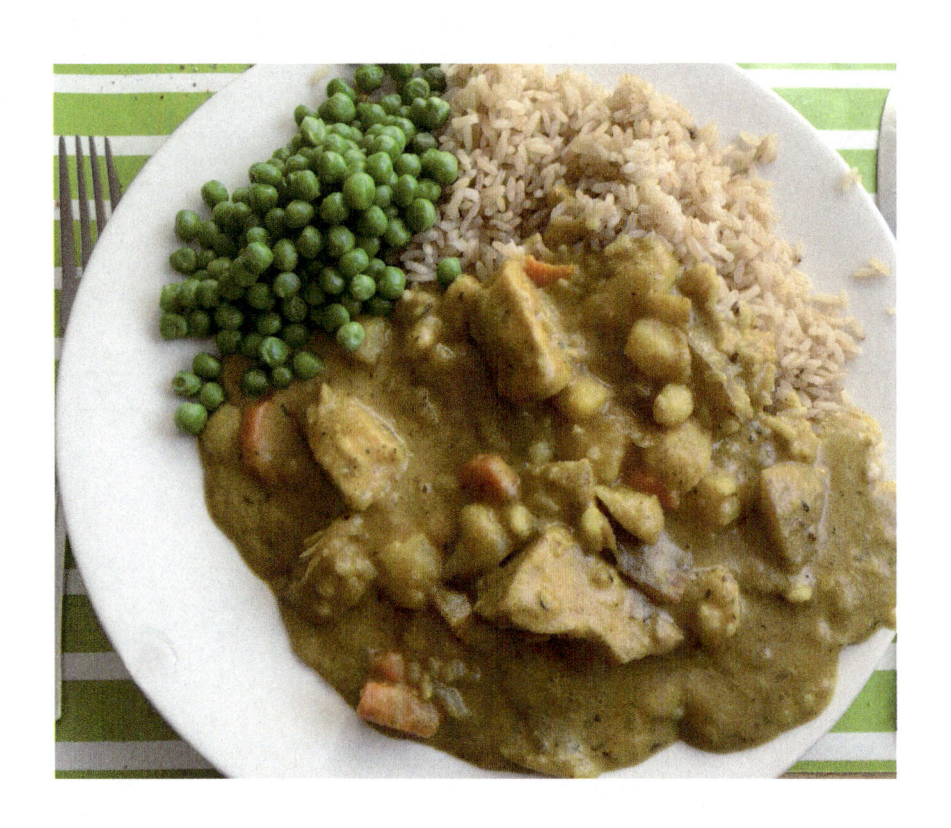

Lentil Chili

| Vegan | Oil-free | WFPB | | Servings: 10 |

The apple cider vinegar in this vegan recipe helps to bring out the flavors and the cocoa powder adds a unique taste.

INGREDIENTS

1 medium yellow onion, chopped

6 cloves garlic, minced

1 medium green bell pepper, seeded and chopped

4 tablespoons (60 ml) chili powder

2 teaspoons (10 ml) oregano

2 teaspoons (10 ml) cumin

1 cup (200g) green lentils

1 cup (200g) red lentils

1 tablespoon (15 ml) apple cider vinegar

6 cups (1.4 L) vegetable broth

2 teaspoons (5 ml) sea salt

1 teaspoon (5 ml) maple syrup

1 teaspoon (5 ml) cocoa powder

1 teaspoon (2.5 ml) black pepper, freshly ground

28 ounces (796g) crushed tomatoes, canned

2 cups (200g) baby spinach, packed, optional

GARNISH (OPTIONAL)

Crushed tortilla chips

Jalapeño slices

DIRECTIONS

1. Add all of the ingredients (with the exception of the baby spinach) to the inner liner of your Instant Pot. Make sure the crushed tomatoes are the last item to go in and DO NOT STIR! Sometimes tomato products that are in contact with the bottom of the inner liner can cause a Burn Notice!
2. Close and lock the lid ensuring that the Pressure Valve is in the Sealing Position.
3. Select the Bean/Chili mode and set the cooking time for 15 minutes.
4. Once cooking time is complete allow a full NPR (Natural Pressure Release).
5. When all of the pressure has been released and the Float Valve has dropped, carefully remove the lid.
6. Add the baby spinach and stir well until the spinach has wilted.
7. Serve immediately with rice, potatoes or pasta.
8. Garnish with crushed tortilla chips and jalapeño slices, if desired.
9. Refrigerate or freeze any leftovers.

Useful Information on total cooking time:

Time to come to pressure: approx. 26 minutes

(Note: we used semi-frozen vegetable broth in this recipe.)

Cooking time: 15 minutes

Full NPR: approx. 30 minutes

Total Instant Pot time: approx. 1 hour, 11 minutes

Nutritional Information per Serving:

Nutritional Information per Serving	
Servings	10
Calories: 192	**Total fat:** 1.06g
Calories from fat: 9 (4%)	Saturated: 0.20g
Total Carbohydrates: 37.03g	Monounsaturated: 0.27g
Dietary Fiber: 7.58g	Polyunsaturated: 0.59g
Sugars: 6.92g	Trans fat: NA
Cholesterol: --	**Sodium:** 1042mg
Protein 11.86g	**Potassium** 649mg
Vitamin A: 2054IU	**Vitamin C:** 21.72mg	**Calcium:** 75mg
Iron: 4.84mg	**Thiamin:** 0.42mg	**Niacin:** 2.50mg
Vitamin B6: 0.47mg	**Magnesium:** 48mg	**Folate:** 210µg

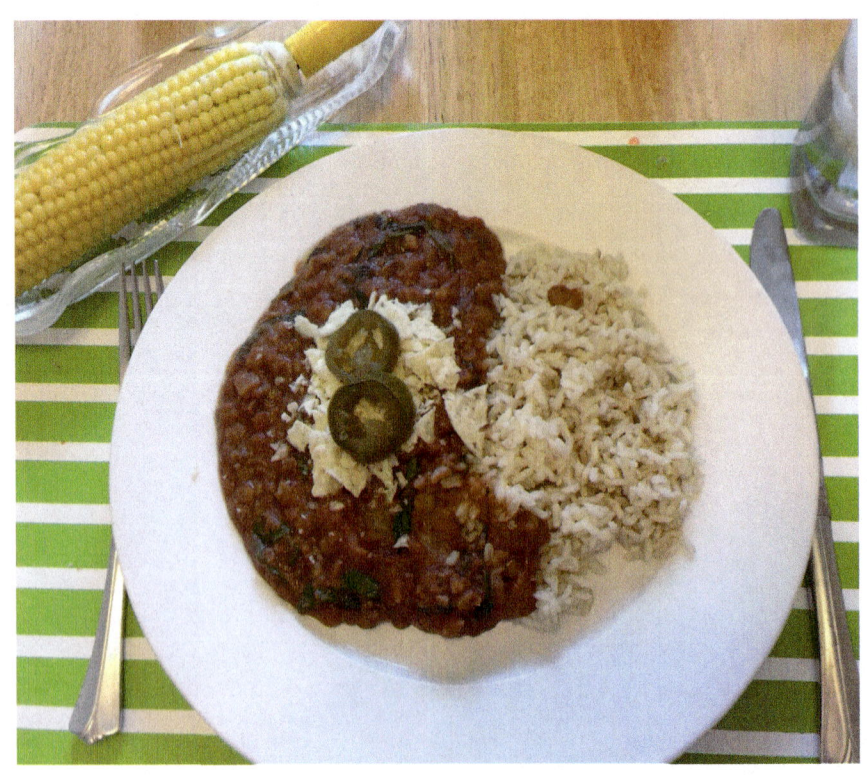

Vicky's Instant Pot Red Beans and Rice

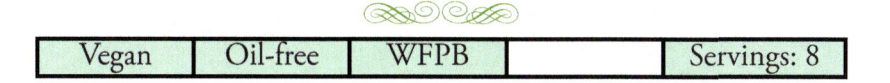

Vegan	Oil-free	WFPB		Servings: 8

This is a super-easy recipe because you get to throw all of the ingredients in together - the beans, the rice and everything else! We used a Bahamian bird pepper because we were able to get them but feel free to use a hot pepper of your choice.

INGREDIENTS

1 large yellow onion, chopped

1 stalk celery, halved and sliced

4 cloves garlic, chopped

1 Bahamian bird pepper (aka Bradley's Bahamian chili pepper), minced with seeds.

Note: If you are able to get this type of pepper, don't be tempted to add more than one. They are small, but they are mighty! (95,000 - 110,000 Scoville Units)

Substitute: if you can't find (or grow) these peppers, look for a small pepper in the same Scoville range.

https://www.cayennediane.com/big-list-of-hot-peppers/

or substitute a hot pepper of your choice depending on your preference.

2 small green peppers, chopped

½ teaspoon (2.5 ml) basil

1 teaspoon (5 ml) black pepper, freshly ground

1½ tablespoons (22.5 ml) cumin

1 teaspoon (5 ml) sea salt

2 cups (450g) brown rice, rinsed

2 cups (400g) dried red beans, rinsed

1 - 14.5 ounce (411g) canned diced tomatoes

6 cups (1.4 L) vegetable broth

DIRECTIONS

1. Add all of the ingredients to the inner liner of your Instant Pot and stir well.
2. Close and lock the lid, ensuring that the Pressure Valve is in the Sealing position.
3. Select the Bean/Chili mode and set the cooking time for 22 minutes.
4. When cooking time is complete, allow a full Natural Pressure Release (this can take 30-45 minutes).
5. Once all the pressure has been released and the Float Valve has dropped, carefully open the lid, stir and serve.
6. Garnish if desired.
7. Optional garnishes: hot sauce, sliced green onion, lime juice

Nutritional Information per Serving:

Nutritional Information per Serving	
Servings 8	
Calories: 397	**Total fat:** 1.99g
Calories from fat: 17 (4%)	Saturated: 0.47g
Total Carbohydrates: 80.13g	Monounsaturated: 0.70g
Dietary Fiber: 10.32g	Polyunsaturated: 0.83g
Sugars: 6.41g	Trans fat: NA
Cholesterol: --	**Sodium:** 817mg
Protein 16.20g	**Potassium** 1165mg
Vitamin A: 630IU	**Vitamin C:** 24.02mg	**Calcium:** 125mg
Iron: 6.02mg	**Thiamin:** 0.67mg	**Niacin:** 3.90mg
Vitamin B6: 0.69mg	**Magnesium:** 183mg	**Folate:** 267µg

Kitchen Sink Cabbage Stew

Vegan	Oil-free	WFPB		Servings: 8

Sometimes you just want to use up some ingredients that you have on hand that lend themselves well to a vegetarian stew.

We like to have a lot of vegetarian options in our cooking and this recipe came together after a survey of the items we had available at the time.

Feel free to make substitutions that work for you.

INGREDIENTS

1 medium onion, chopped

3 cloves garlic, minced

2 ribs celery, chopped

2 carrots, peeled and chopped

1 medium yam, peeled and chunked

1½ cups (250g) black beans, cooked (may be frozen)

1 small head of green cabbage chopped into large chunks

½ small head cauliflower, chunked

1½ cups (350 ml) tomato sauce

15 ounces (440 ml) canned diced tomatoes, with liquid

2 cups (480 ml) vegetable broth, preferably homemade

2 teaspoons (10 ml) sea salt

1 teaspoon (5 ml) black pepper, freshly ground

1½ teaspoons (7.5 ml) dried oregano

1 teaspoon (5 ml) fennel seeds

¼ teaspoon (1.25 ml) crushed red pepper flakes

1 tablespoon (15 ml) vegan Worcestershire sauce

2 cups (200g) baby spinach, packed

DIRECTIONS

1. Add all of the ingredients, with the exception of the spinach, to the inner liner of your Instant Pot.
2. Close and lock the lid ensuring that the Pressure Valve is in the Sealing position.
3. Select the Soup/Broth mode and set the cooking time for 4 minutes.
4. Once cooking time is complete, allow a Natural Pressure Release for 10 minutes and then release the rest of the pressure by carefully turning the Pressure Valve from Sealing to Venting.
5. Once all of the pressure has been released and the Float Valve has dropped, carefully remove the lid.
6. Stir in the baby spinach and allow it to wilt.
7. Serve immediately or allow to cool and refrigerate or freeze for later use.

Nutritional Information per Serving:

Nutritional Information per Serving		
Servings 8		
Calories: 172	**Total fat:** 1.72g	
Calories from fat: 15 (8%)	Saturated: 0.42g	
Total Carbohydrates: 35.07g	Monounsaturated: 0.64g	
Dietary Fiber: 10.07g	Polyunsaturated: 0.66g	
Sugars: 8.08g	Trans fat: NA	
Cholesterol: --	**Sodium:** 1428mg	
Protein 7.16g	**Potassium** 988mg	
Vitamin A: 4172IU	**Vitamin C:** 72.09mg	**Calcium:** 123mg
Iron: 3.21mg	**Thiamin:** 0.25mg	**Niacin:** 2.10mg
Vitamin B6: 0.41mg	**Magnesium:** 63mg	**Folate:** 126µg

Red Lentil & Greens Curry

Vegan	Oil-free	WFPB		Servings: 4

You can include greens of your choice in this tasty curry - baby kale, baby spinach, beet greens - it's up to you. We've tried it with all of them.

INGREDIENTS

½ medium yellow onion, chopped

½ medium red onion, chopped

1 stalk celery, sliced

4 cloves garlic, minced

2 large carrots, chopped

1 large green bell pepper, chopped

2 tablespoons (30 ml) curry powder

1 teaspoon (5 ml) ground ginger

1 teaspoon (5 ml) turmeric

1 teaspoon (5 ml) sea salt, or to taste

1⅓ cups (265g) red lentils

¾ cup (180 ml) coconut milk

4 cups (400g) baby spinach, packed, or substitute beet greens or baby kale

DIRECTIONS

1. Add all of the ingredients to the inner pot of your Instant Pot with the exception of the coconut milk and greens.
2. Close and lock the lid ensuring the Pressure Valve is in the Sealing position.

3. Select the Pressure Cook/Manual setting and set cooking time for 10 minutes.
4. Once cooking time is complete, allow a 10-minute Natural Pressure Release (NPR) and then release the rest of the pressure by carefully turning the Pressure Valve from Sealing to Venting.
5. Once all of the pressure has been released and the Float Valve has dropped, carefully remove the lid.
6. Add the coconut milk and greens of your choice (whatever greens you have chosen will wilt pretty quickly).
7. Stir well and serve immediately over rice (or starch of your choice).
8. Leftovers freeze well.

Nutritional Information per Serving:

Nutritional Information per Serving		
Servings 4		
Calories: 377	**Total fat:** 9.72g	
Calories from fat: 87 (23%)	Saturated: 8.25g	
Total Carbohydrates: 56.63g	Monounsaturated: 0.80g	
Dietary Fiber: 12.05g	Polyunsaturated: 0.67g	
Sugars: 7.15g	Trans fat: NA	
Cholesterol: --	**Sodium:** 658mg	
Protein 19.51g	**Potassium** 1060mg	
Vitamin A: 9076IU	**Vitamin C:** 51.29mg	**Calcium:** 116mg
Iron: 7.95mg	**Thiamin:** 0.67mg	**Niacin:** 2.99mg
Vitamin B6: 0.67mg	**Magnesium:** 98mg	**Folate:** 400µg

INSTANT POT ITALIAN BEAN CASSEROLE

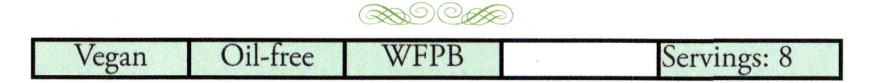

| Vegan | Oil-free | WFPB | | Servings: 8 |

You can use any kind of pasta you choose for this recipe. We used elbow macaroni. If you use spaghetti or some other long noodle, be sure to break it up into smaller pieces.

This nutritious casserole is high in both protein and fiber, thanks to the beans, and has no added fat.

We love one pot meals!

INGREDIENTS

4 cups (950 ml) vegetable broth

8 ounces (225g) pasta, your choice

2 cups (125g) Great Northern beans, canned or home cooked

2 cups (125g) small red beans, canned or home cooked

1 medium yellow onion, chopped

1 stalk celery, chopped

1 medium zucchini, chopped

3 cloves garlic, minced

1 tablespoon (15 ml) Italian seasoning

½ teaspoon (2.5 ml) black pepper, freshly ground

1½ teaspoons (7.5 ml) sea salt

28 ounces (795g) diced tomatoes, canned

DIRECTIONS

1. Place all of the ingredients in the inner liner of your Instant Pot in the order given and DO NOT STIR! (The reason we're not going

to stir this is because if the tomatoes are directly on the bottom you could get the dreaded BURN notice. Don't worry, everything will cook just fine if you don't stir it.)

2. Close and lock the lid ensuring the Pressure Valve is in the Sealing position.
3. Select the Pressure Cook/Manual setting and set the cooking time for 4 minutes.
4. Once cooking time is complete, do a QR (Quick Release). (that means carefully turning the Pressure valve from Sealing to Venting)
5. When all the pressure has been released and the Float Valve has dropped, carefully remove the lid.
6. Give it a good stir and serve immediately or refrigerate or freeze for later use.

Nutritional Information per Serving:

Nutritional Information per Serving			
Servings	8		
Calories: 467		**Total fat:** 1.34g	
Calories from fat: 12 (2%)		Saturated: 0.39g	
Total Carbohydrates: 89.84g		Monounsaturated: 0.16g	
Dietary Fiber: 19.98g		Polyunsaturated: 0.79g	
Sugars: 9.46g		Trans fat: NA	
Cholesterol: --		**Sodium:** 917mg	
Protein 26.34g		**Potassium** 1732mg	
Vitamin A: 560IU	**Vitamin C:** 19.64mg	**Calcium:** 181mg
Iron: 8.23mg	**Thiamin:** 0.92mg	**Niacin:** 5.30mg
Vitamin B6: 0.65mg	**Magnesium:** 193mg	**Folate:** 494µg

Spicy Lentils with Potato and Spinach

Vegan	Oil-free	WFPB		Servings: 4

INGREDIENTS

½ cup (100g) green lentils, soaked for at least one hour and rinsed

4 cloves garlic, minced

1 tablespoon (15 ml) ginger, minced

1 medium jalapeño, chopped, seeds removed

2 cups (400g) diced tomatoes

½ teaspoon (2.5 ml) garam masala

¼ teaspoon (1.25 ml) cinnamon

¼ teaspoon (1.25 ml) cardamom

½ teaspoon (2.5 ml) turmeric

4 small red potatoes, cubed

1 teaspoon (5 ml) sea salt

1½ cups (350 ml) vegetable broth

1 cup (100g) baby spinach, packed, can substitute other greens like beet greens or kale

DIRECTIONS

1. Put all of the ingredients in the inner liner of your Instant Pot and stir well.
2. Close and lock the lid, ensuring the Pressure Valve is in the Sealing Position.
3. Select Pressure Cook/Manual and set the cooking time to 3 minutes.

4. When cooking time is complete, allow a full NPR (Natural Pressure Release). This means just let your Instant Pot sit until the Float Valve drops on its own.
5. When all of the pressure has been released and the Float Valve has dropped, carefully remove the lid and stir.
6. Serve immediately or refrigerate or freeze for later use.

Nutritional Information per Serving:

Nutritional Information per Serving		
Servings 4		
Calories: 263	**Total fat:** 0.66g	
Calories from fat: 5 (2%)	Saturated: 0.17g	
Total Carbohydrates: 55.22g	Monounsaturated: 0.13g	
Dietary Fiber: 8.20g	Polyunsaturated: 0.36g	
Sugars: 8.81g	Trans fat: NA	
Cholesterol: --	**Sodium:** 1036mg	
Protein 11.72g	**Potassium** 1360mg	
Vitamin A: 1212IU	**Vitamin C:** 36.84mg	**Calcium:** 79mg
Iron: 4.91mg	**Thiamin:** 0.40mg	**Niacin:** 4.56mg
Vitamin B6: 0.68mg	**Magnesium:** 85mg	**Folate:** 182µg

Eggplant and Sweet Potato Curry

| Vegan | Oil-free | WFPB | | Servings: 8 |

INGREDIENTS

¾ cup (150g) green lentils

2 cups (475 ml) vegetable broth, preferably homemade

1 medium yellow onion, chopped

4 cloves garlic, minced

1 tablespoon (15 ml) ginger, minced

½ teaspoon (2.5 ml) turmeric

1 tablespoon (15 ml) curry powder

1 teaspoon (5 ml) cumin

28 ounces (795g) diced tomatoes, canned

4 cups (1 Kg) eggplant, chopped

4 cups (600g) sweet potato, chopped

1 teaspoon (5 ml) sea salt

2 cups (200g) baby spinach, washed and packed

½ cup (120 ml) coconut milk

DIRECTIONS

1. Prepare all the ingredients per the list of ingredients.
2. Add all the ingredients to the inner pot of the Instant Pot, with the exception of the spinach and the coconut milk.
3. Close and lock the lid of the Instant Pot, ensuring that the Pressure Valve is in the Sealing Position.
4. Select the Pressure Cook/Manual setting and set the cooking time for 4 minutes.

5. When cooking time is complete, allow a 10-minute Natural Pressure Release, then carefully turn the Pressure Valve from Sealing to Venting to release any remaining pressure.
6. Once all the pressure has been released and the Float Valve has dropped, carefully remove the lid.
7. Carefully remove the inner pot to a heatproof surface.
8. Add the spinach and coconut milk. Stir well and serve with rice and/or your favorite side dishes.
9. This recipe freezes well if you want to freeze any leftovers.

Useful Information on total cooking time:

Time to come to pressure: approx. 18-23 minutes

Cooking time: 4 minutes

NPR: 10 minutes

QR: time for pressure to release: 5-8 minutes

Total Instant Pot time: approx. 37-50 minutes

Nutritional Information per Serving:

Nutritional Information per Serving		
Servings	8	
Calories: 239	**Total fat:** 3.52g	
Calories from fat: 31 (13%)	Saturated: 2.82g	
Total Carbohydrates: 46.30g	Monounsaturated: 0.32g	
Dietary Fiber: 9.13g	Polyunsaturated: 0.37g	
Sugars: 7.74g	Trans fat: NA	
Cholesterol: --	**Sodium:** 630mg	
Protein 8.59g	**Potassium** 1243mg	
Vitamin A: 1165IU	**Vitamin C:** 27.43mg	**Calcium:** 79mg
Iron: 4.24mg	**Thiamin:** 0.34mg	**Niacin:** 2.62mg
Vitamin B6: 0.55mg	**Magnesium:** 68mg	**Folate:** 144µg

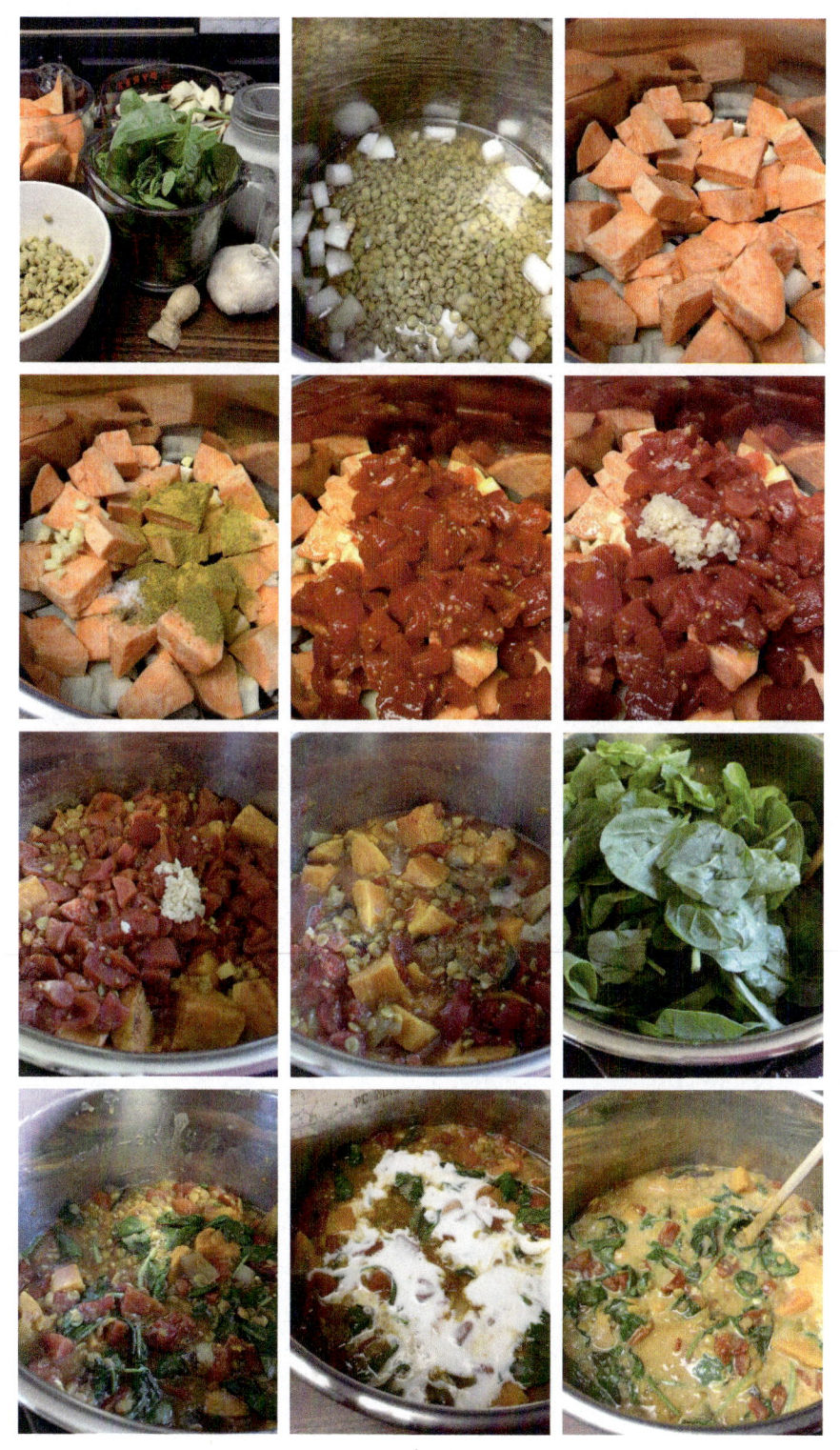

Lentil Stuffed Peppers

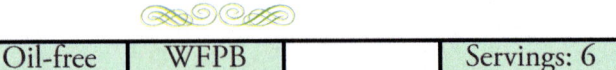

| Vegan | Oil-free | WFPB | | Servings: 6 |

This is a "some assembly required" recipe for Lentil Stuffed Peppers with only part of it being cooked in the Instant Pot.

PREPARE THE LENTILS

1 cup (200g) green lentils

2 cups (475 ml) vegetable broth, preferably homemade

PREPARE THE COUSCOUS

¾ cup (165g) couscous, preferably whole wheat

1 cup (240 ml) vegetable broth, preferably homemade

REST OF THE INGREDIENTS

3 large bell peppers, halved lengthwise, your choice of color

½ medium yellow onion, minced

1 stalk celery, minced

4 cloves garlic, minced

½ cup (120 ml) crushed tomato

1 tablespoon (15 ml) poultry seasoning

1 tablespoon (15 ml) Italian seasoning

1 teaspoon (5 ml) sea salt

1 teaspoon (5 ml) black pepper, freshly ground

COOK THE LENTILS:

Note: Make the lentils early in the day and allow to cool.

INSTANT POT DIRECTIONS

1. Place 1 cup (240 ml) of water and the trivet in the inner pot of the Instant Pot.
2. Place 1 cup (200g) of lentils and 2 cups (475 ml) of vegetable broth in an oven-safe dish and place on the trivet in the Instant Pot.
3. Close and lock the lid, ensuring that the Pressure Valve is in the Sealing position.
4. Select the Bean/Chili mode and set the cooking time for 15 minutes.
5. When cooking time is complete, allow a full Natural Pressure Release (NPR).
6. Once all the pressure has been released and the Float Valve has dropped, carefully remove the lid.
7. Remove the dish holding the lentils to a heatproof surface and allow the lentils to cool.

COOK THE COUSCOUS:

1. In a small saucepan, bring the vegetable broth to a boil.
2. Add the couscous. Stir and cover. Turn off the heat and let the couscous sit for 5 minutes.

MAKE THE FILLING:

1. Mix together the cooked lentils, cooked couscous, onions, garlic, celery, crushed tomatoes and spices.
2. Fill the peppers with the mixture and place in a lightly greased baking dish.
3. Cover and bake at 350°F for 30 minutes. Uncover and bake for an additional 15 minutes.
4. Remove from oven and serve with a sauce and side dishes of your choice.

Nutritional Information per Serving:

Nutritional Information per Serving		
Servings	6	
Calories: 235		**Total fat:** 0.62g
Calories from fat: 5 (2%)		Saturated: 0.17g
Total Carbohydrates: 46.98g		Monounsaturated: 0.12g
Dietary Fiber: 7.21g		Polyunsaturated: 0.34g
Sugars: 5.11g		Trans fat: NA
Cholesterol: --	**Sodium:** 715mg	
Protein 12.17g	**Potassium** 525mg	
Vitamin A: 693IU	**Vitamin C:** 70.97mg	**Calcium:** 64mg
Iron: 3.56mg	**Thiamin:** 0.38mg	**Niacin:** 2.35mg
Vitamin B6: 0.47mg	**Magnesium:** 43mg	**Folate:** 176µg

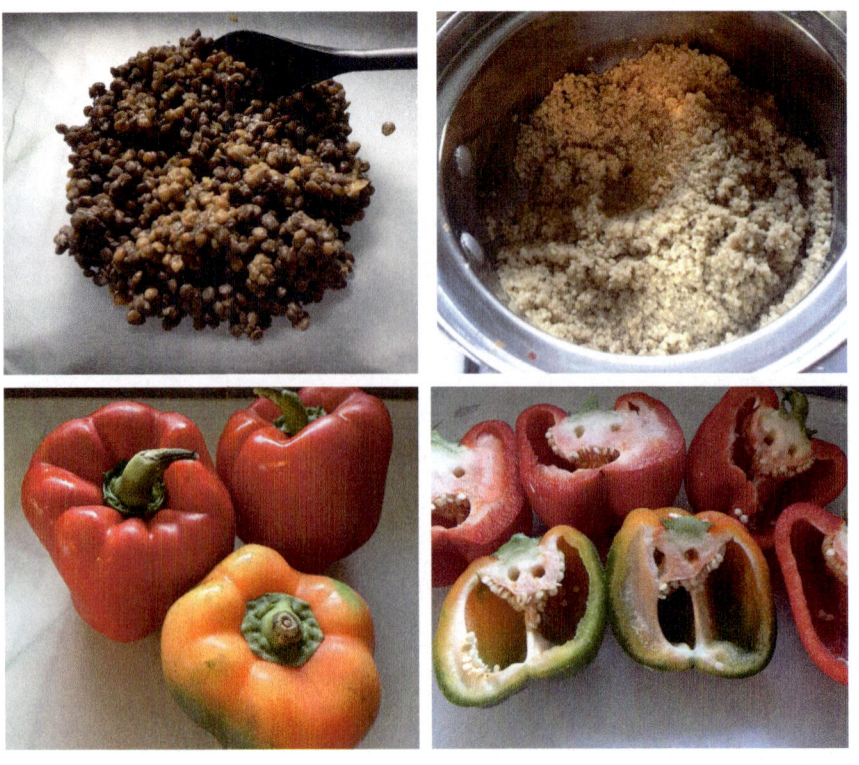

53

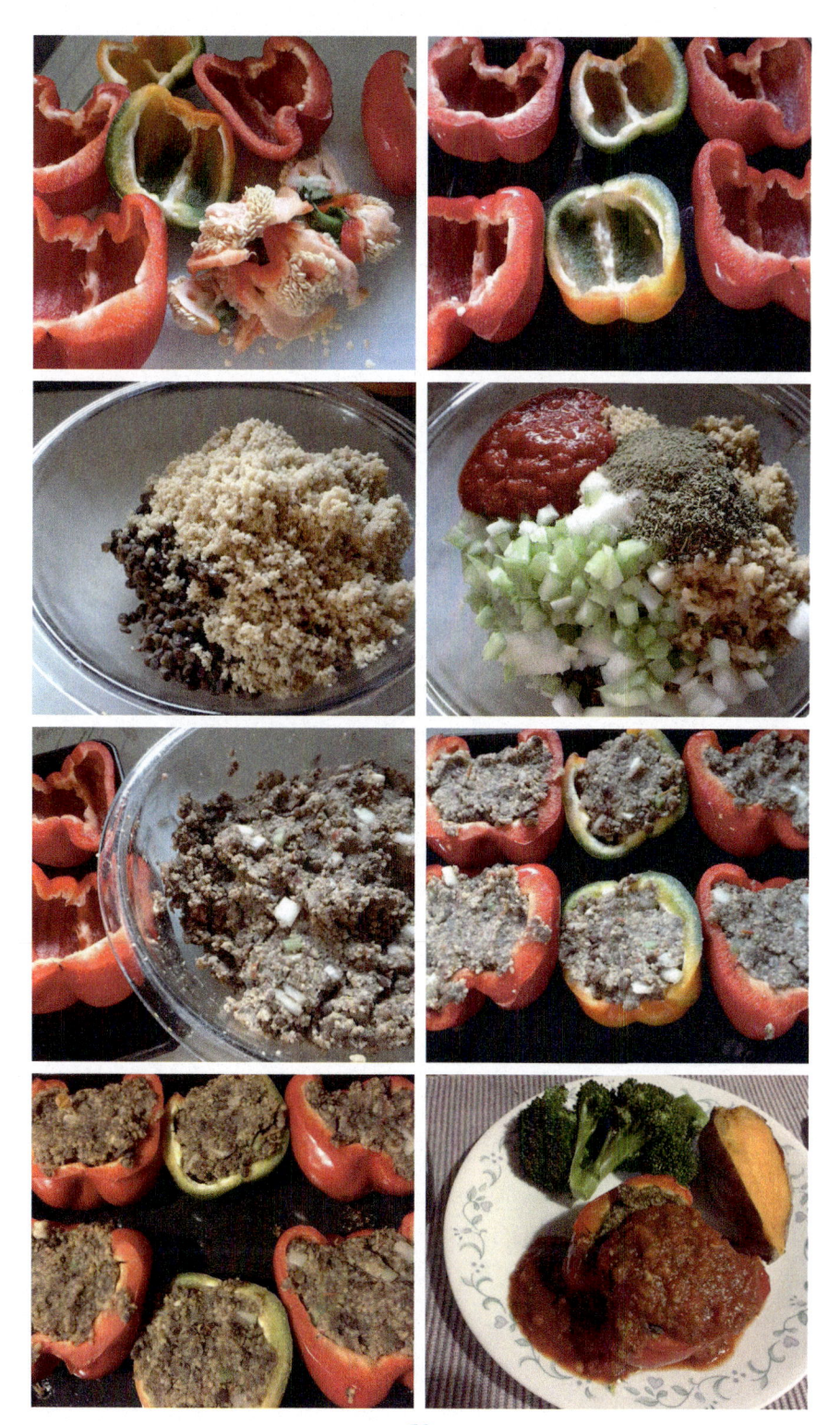

Detox Cabbage Stew

| Vegan | Oil-free | WFPB | | Servings: 10 |

There is lots of good stuff in this stew to help you detox. And, it's super low in calories, too!

We used a 6-quart Instant Pot for this recipe and that totally filled it up to the Max line, so if you've got an 8-quart, it would work well in that, too. And, in the 8-quart, you could even add more veggies without altering the calories much.

INGREDIENTS

4 cups (950 ml) vegetable broth

½ large cabbage, quartered and sliced

1 large yellow onion, quartered and sliced

2 stalks celery, chopped

3 large carrots, chopped

1½ cups (245g) chickpeas, canned and drained or home cooked

8 medium radishes, halved or quartered, depending on size

5 cloves garlic, chopped

3 tablespoons (45 ml) apple cider vinegar

1½ tablespoons (22.5 ml) lemon juice

2 teaspoons (10 ml) sea salt

1 teaspoon (5 ml) black pepper, freshly ground

1½ tablespoons (22.5 ml) Herbes de Provence, or Italian seasoning

½ teaspoon (2.5 ml) red pepper flakes, optional

28 ounces (795g) diced tomatoes

2 cups (200g) baby spinach, packed

DIRECTIONS

1. Prepare all of the ingredients per the ingredient list.
2. Add all ingredients, with the exception of the spinach, to the inner pot of your Instant Pot, in the order given and DO NOT STIR. The reason you don't want to stir it is so that you don't get the tomatoes on the bottom, which could cause a BURN notice!
3. Close and lock the lid, ensuring the Pressure Valve is in the Sealing position.
4. Select Soup/Broth mode and set the cooking time for 5 minutes.
5. Once the cooking time is complete, allow a 10-minute NPR (Natural Pressure Release). Hint: allowing a 10-minute NPR allows the contents to "settle down" a bit before you release the pressure, so you're less likely to get anything spewing out of the Pressure Valve.
6. When the 10 minutes is up, release the rest of the pressure by carefully turning the Pressure Valve from Sealing to Venting.
7. When all of the pressure has been released and the Float Valve has dropped, carefully remove the lid.
8. Add the spinach and stir until it is wilted and incorporated into the stew.
9. Carefully remove the inner liner to a heatproof surface, give the stew another good stir and serve immediately or refrigerate or freeze for later use.

Useful Information on total cooking time:

Time to come to pressure: approx. 28 minutes

Cooking time: 5 minutes

NPR: 10 minutes

QR: time for pressure to release: approx. 5 minutes

Total Instant Pot time: approx. 48 minutes

Nutritional Information per Serving:

Nutritional Information per Serving	
Servings 10	
Calories: 101	Total fat: 0.85g
Calories from fat: 7 (7%)	Saturated: 0.16g
Total Carbohydrates: 20.92g	Monounsaturated: 0.21g
Dietary Fiber: 6.26g	Polyunsaturated: 0.48g
Sugars: 8.33g	Trans fat: NA
Cholesterol: --	Sodium: 976mg
Protein 4.71g	Potassium 579mg

Vitamin A:	4714IU	Vitamin C:	36.61mg	Calcium:	99mg
Iron:	2.33mg	Thiamin:	0.13mg	Niacin:	1.53mg
Vitamin B6:	0.46mg	Magnesium:	45mg	Folate:	71μg

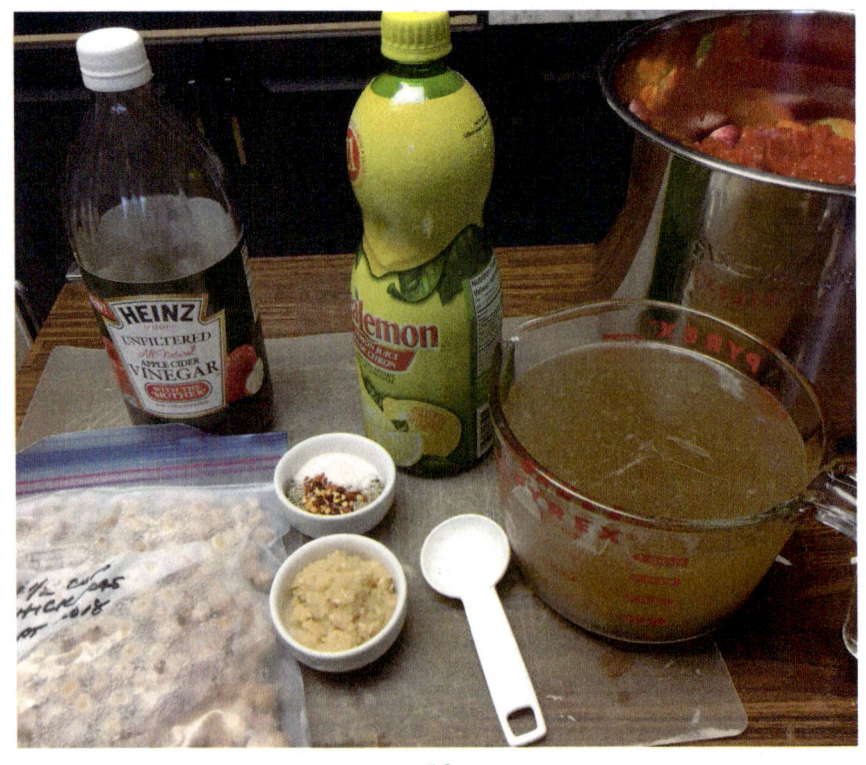

57

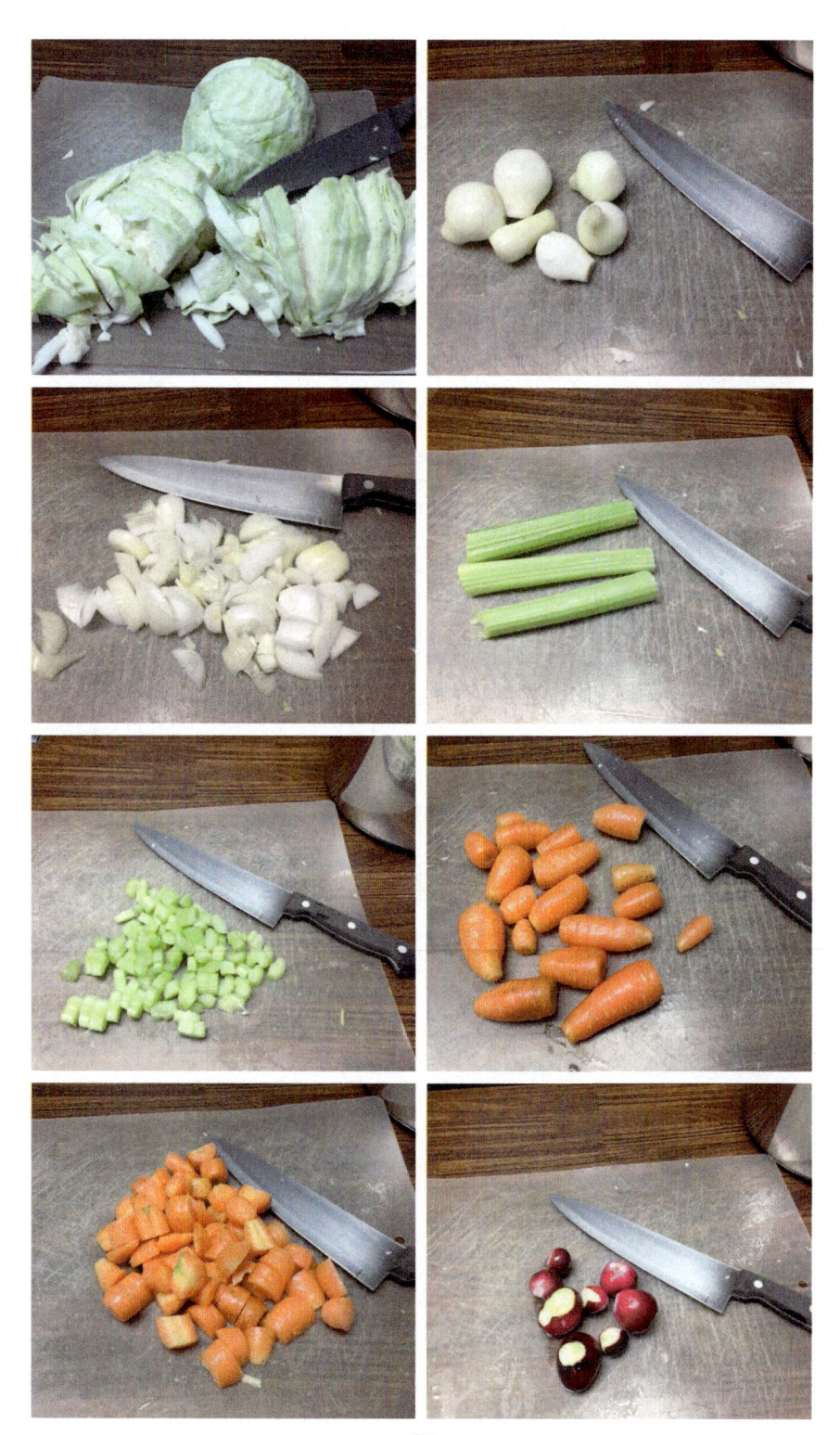

58

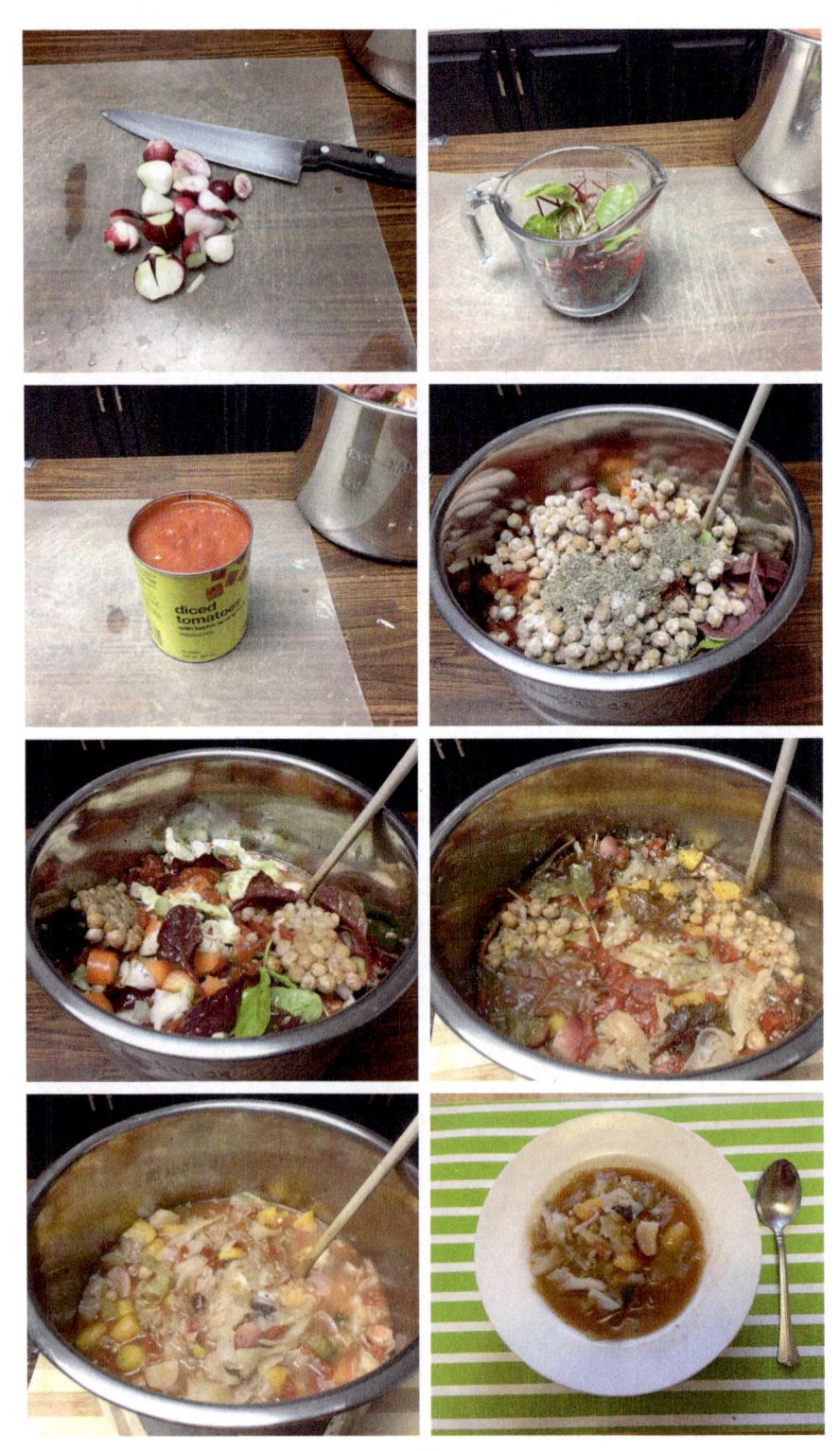

Sicilian-Style Fava Beans

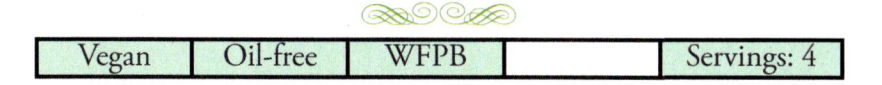

| Vegan | Oil-free | WFPB | | Servings: 4 |

When buying the dried fava beans, always be sure to purchase the ones that have already been shelled. We neglected to do that once and had to spend ages shelling the beans. We learned our lesson and haven't made that mistake again.

These beans are lovely served with some rice or pasta, a small salad, some hearty bread to mop up any leftover juices and, of course, a glass of your favorite red wine.

INGREDIENTS

2 cups (240g) dried split fava beans

½ cup (120 ml) red wine

4 cups (950 ml) vegetable broth

1 medium yellow onion, diced

4 cloves garlic, minced

1 stalk celery, diced

1 tablespoon (15 ml) dried oregano

1 tablespoon (15 ml) dried basil

½ teaspoon (2.5 ml) fennel seed

1 tablespoon (15 ml) black pepper, freshly ground

½ teaspoon (2.5 ml) crushed red pepper flakes, optional

1 bay leaf

2 cups (400g) diced tomatoes, fresh or canned

1½ teaspoons (7.5 ml) sea salt

DIRECTIONS:

1. Combine all ingredients in the inner liner of your Instant Pot in the order given. DO NOT STIR! (Note: the reason we don't stir this is because tomatoes can often give you the dreaded "Burn" notice. Also, we want to make sure that the beans are submerged in the vegetable broth.)
2. Close and lock the lid ensuring the Pressure Valve is in the Sealing Position.
3. Select the Beans/Chili setting and set the cooking time for 22 minutes.
4. When cooking time is complete allow a full Natural Pressure Release (NPR). That means allowing the pot to just sit until the Float Valve drops on its own. (This can take quite some time – 30 minutes or more.)
5. When the Float Valve has dropped, carefully remove the lid and then remove the inner liner to a heatproof surface.
6. Give it a good stir and serve immediately over rice or pasta.

   Note: Any leftovers freeze well.

Nutritional Information per Serving:

Nutritional Information per Serving		
Servings 8		
Calories: 180	**Total fat:** 0.69g	
Calories from fat: 6 (3%)	Saturated: 0.17g	
Total Carbohydrates: 31.65g	Monounsaturated: 0.18g	
Dietary Fiber: 11.73g	Polyunsaturated: 0.34g	
Sugars: 6.65g	Trans fat: NA	
Cholesterol: --	**Sodium:** 836mg	
Protein 11.42g	**Potassium** 680mg	
Vitamin A: 508IU	**Vitamin C:** 7.99mg	**Calcium:** 98mg
Iron: 4.34mg	**Thiamin:** 0.26mg	**Niacin:** 1.97mg
Vitamin B6: 0.30mg	**Magnesium:** 95mg	**Folate:** 175μg

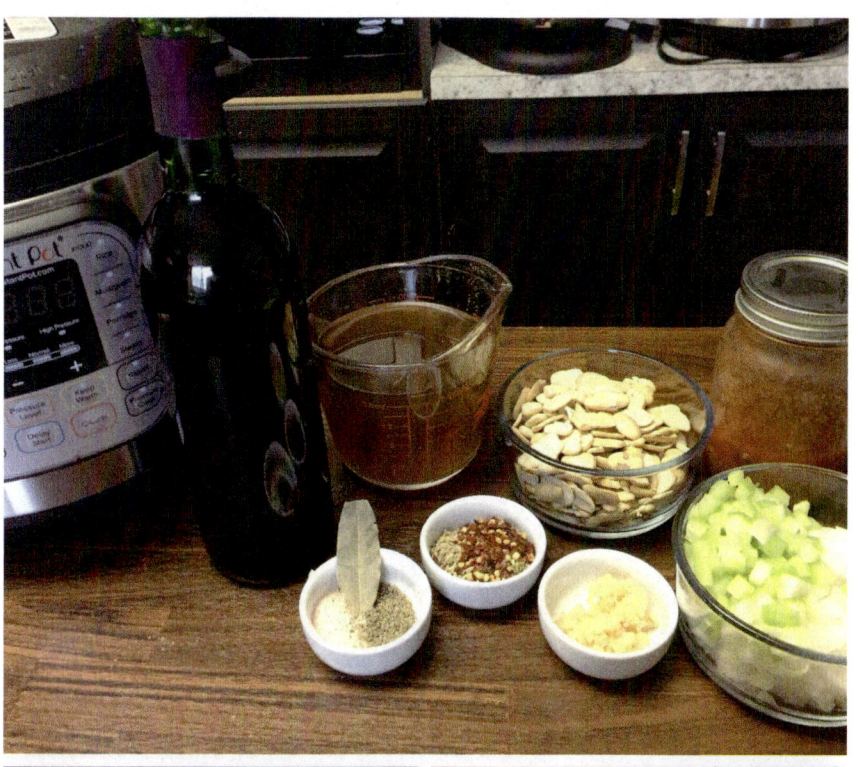

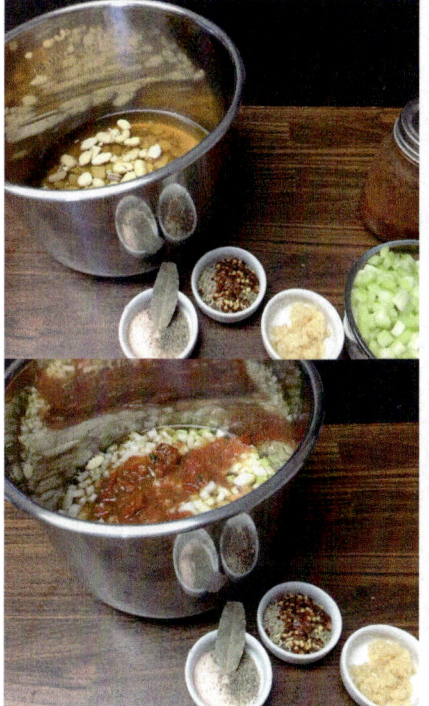

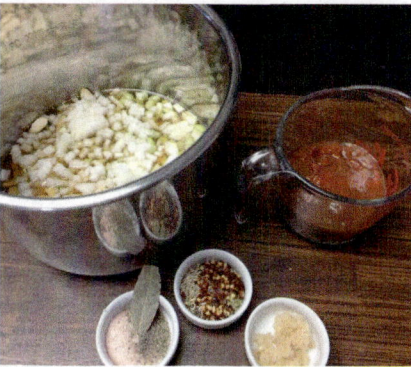

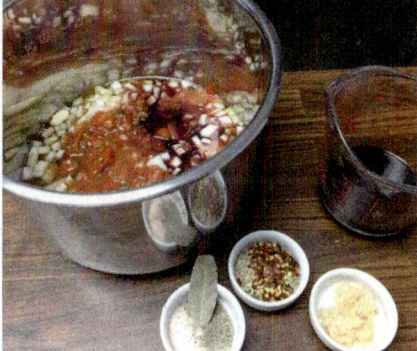

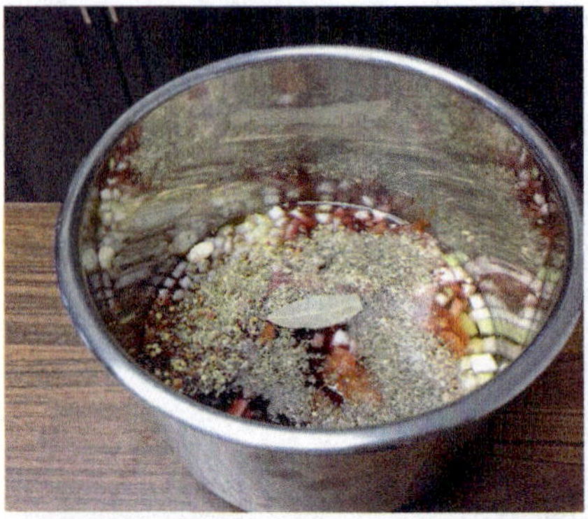

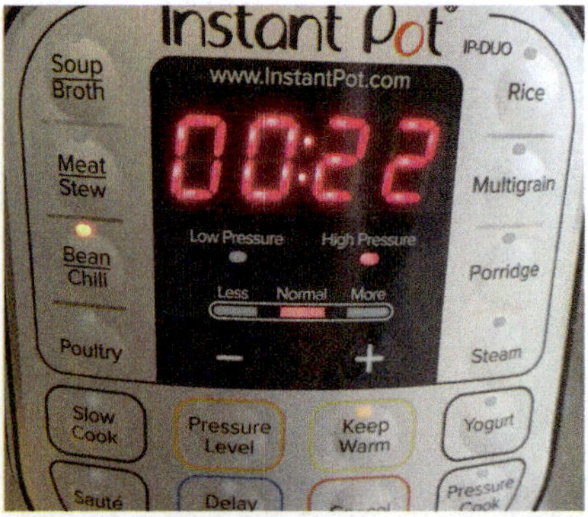
Instant Pot
IP-DUO
www.InstantPot.com
00:22
Soup Broth
Meat Stew
Bean Chili
Poultry
Rice
Multigrain
Porridge
Steam
Low Pressure
High Pressure
Less
Normal
More
Slow Cook
Pressure Level
Keep Warm
Yogurt
Sauté
Delay

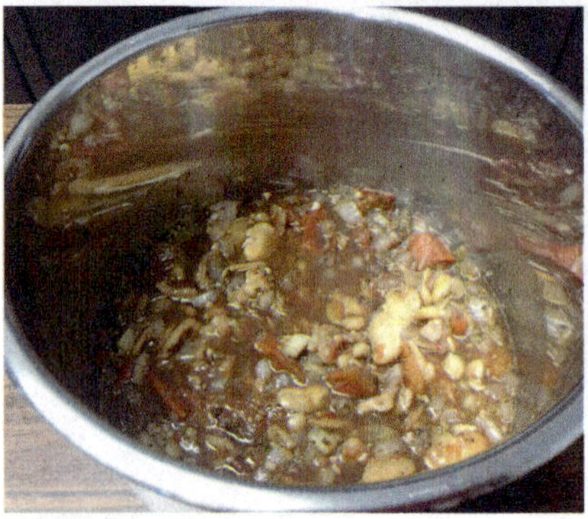

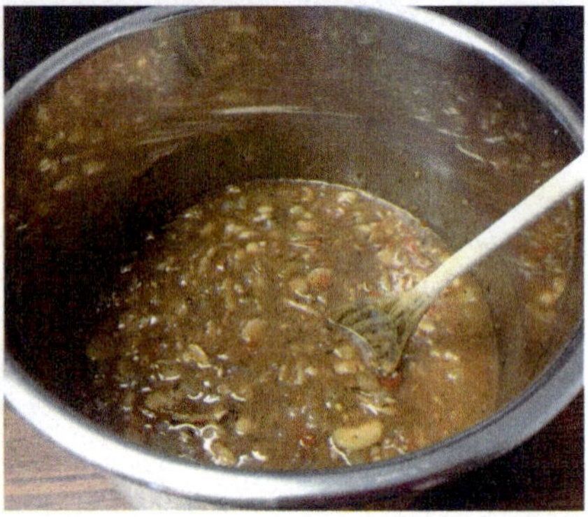

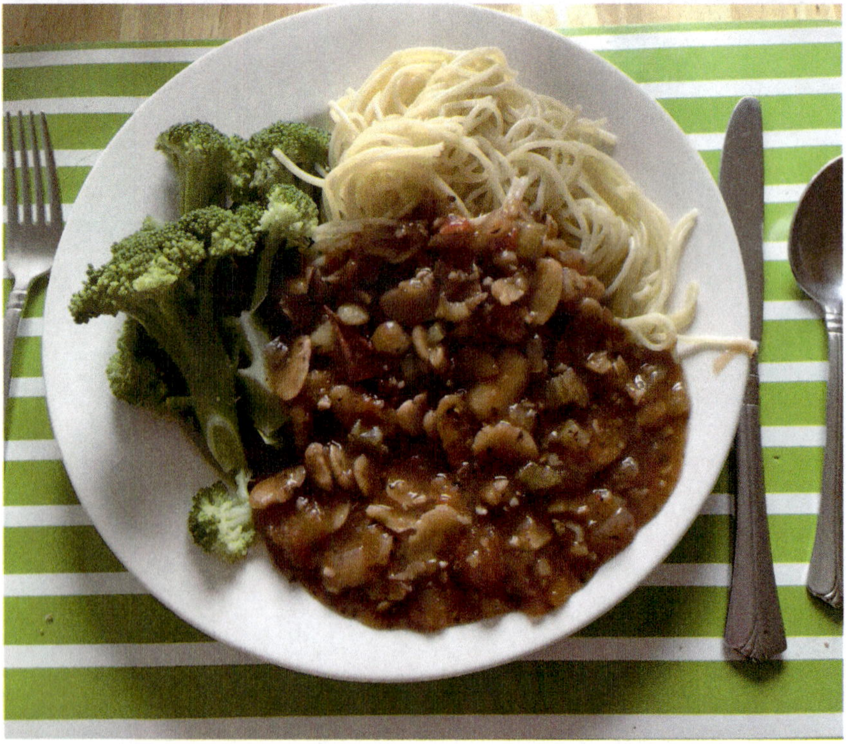

CREMINI POT ROAST

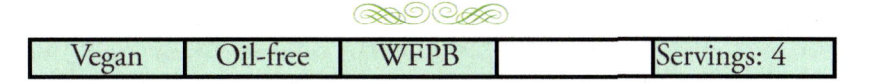

| Vegan | Oil-free | WFPB | | Servings: 4 |

Who says a pot roast has to include meat?

This recipe features hearty Cremini (baby bella) mushrooms as the basis for this healthy pot roast.

Serve it with a side-dish of your choice, and a crusty bread to help soak up some of the gravy!

And, if you wish, pair it with your favorite wine.

INGREDIENTS

4 medium red potatoes, chunked

1 pound (454g) Cremini mushrooms, halved

4 medium carrots, chunked

2 large parsnips, chunked

1 large yellow onion, sliced

4 cloves garlic, minced

2 teaspoons (10 ml) thyme

3 cups (700 ml) vegetable broth, divided

½ cup (120 ml) dry red wine

3 tablespoons (45 ml) tomato paste

2 tablespoons (30 ml) vegan Worcestershire sauce

2 tablespoons (30 ml) cornstarch

sea salt, to taste

black pepper, freshly ground, to taste

DIRECTIONS

1. Prepare all the ingredients per the list of ingredients.
2. Add all the ingredients to the inner pot of the Instant Pot, reserving a couple of tablespoons of the vegetable broth to mix with the cornstarch later.
3. Close and lock the lid of the Instant Pot, ensuring that the Pressure Valve is in the Sealing Position.
4. Select the Pressure Cook/Manual button and set the cooking time for 2 minutes.
5. Once the cooking time is complete, allow a 4-minute Natural Pressure Release, then carefully turn the Pressure Valve from Sealing to Venting to release any remaining pressure.
6. Once all the pressure has been released and the Float Valve has dropped, carefully remove the lid, turn the Instant Pot off and then select the Sauté mode.
7. Mix the cornstarch with 2 tablespoons of vegetable broth to make a pourable slurry.
8. With the content still bubbling, slowly pour in the cornstarch slurry, stirring constantly until the gravy has thickened. Add salt and pepper to taste. Turn off the Instant Pot.
9. Serve immediately with your favorite side dish(es).

Note: This recipe freezes well if you have any leftovers.

Useful Information on total cooking time:

Time to come to pressure: approx. 18 minutes
Cooking time: 2 minutes
NPR: 4 minutes
QR: time for pressure to release: 1-2 minutes
Total Instant Pot time: approx. 25-26 minutes

Nutritional Information per Serving:

Nutritional Information per Serving		
Servings 4		
Calories: 327	**Total fat:** 0.48g	
Calories from fat: 4 (1%)	Saturated: 0.14g	
Total Carbohydrates: 69.50g	Monounsaturated: 0.10g	
Dietary Fiber: 9.77g	Polyunsaturated: 0.24g	
Sugars: 14.95g	Trans fat: NA	
Cholesterol: --	**Sodium:** 580mg	
Protein 9.09g	**Potassium** 2153mg	
Vitamin A: 10799IU	**Vitamin C:** 42.42mg	**Calcium:** 115mg
Iron: 4.14mg	**Thiamin:** 0.35mg	**Niacin:** 8.68mg
Vitamin B6: 0.72mg	**Magnesium:** 97mg	**Folate:** 136µg

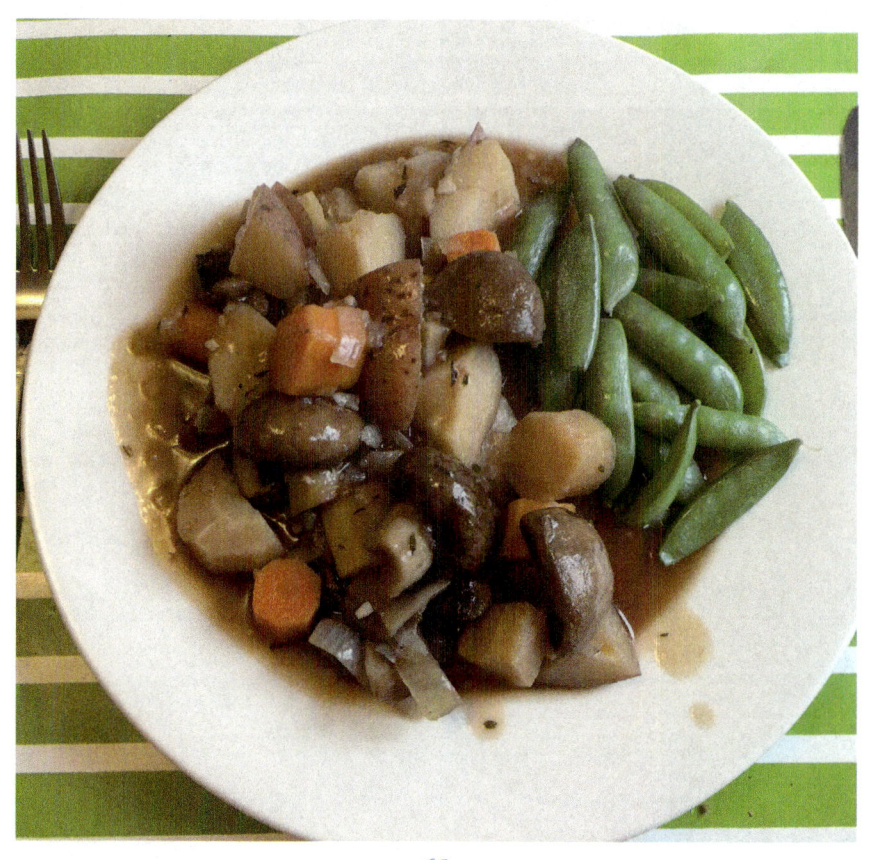

66

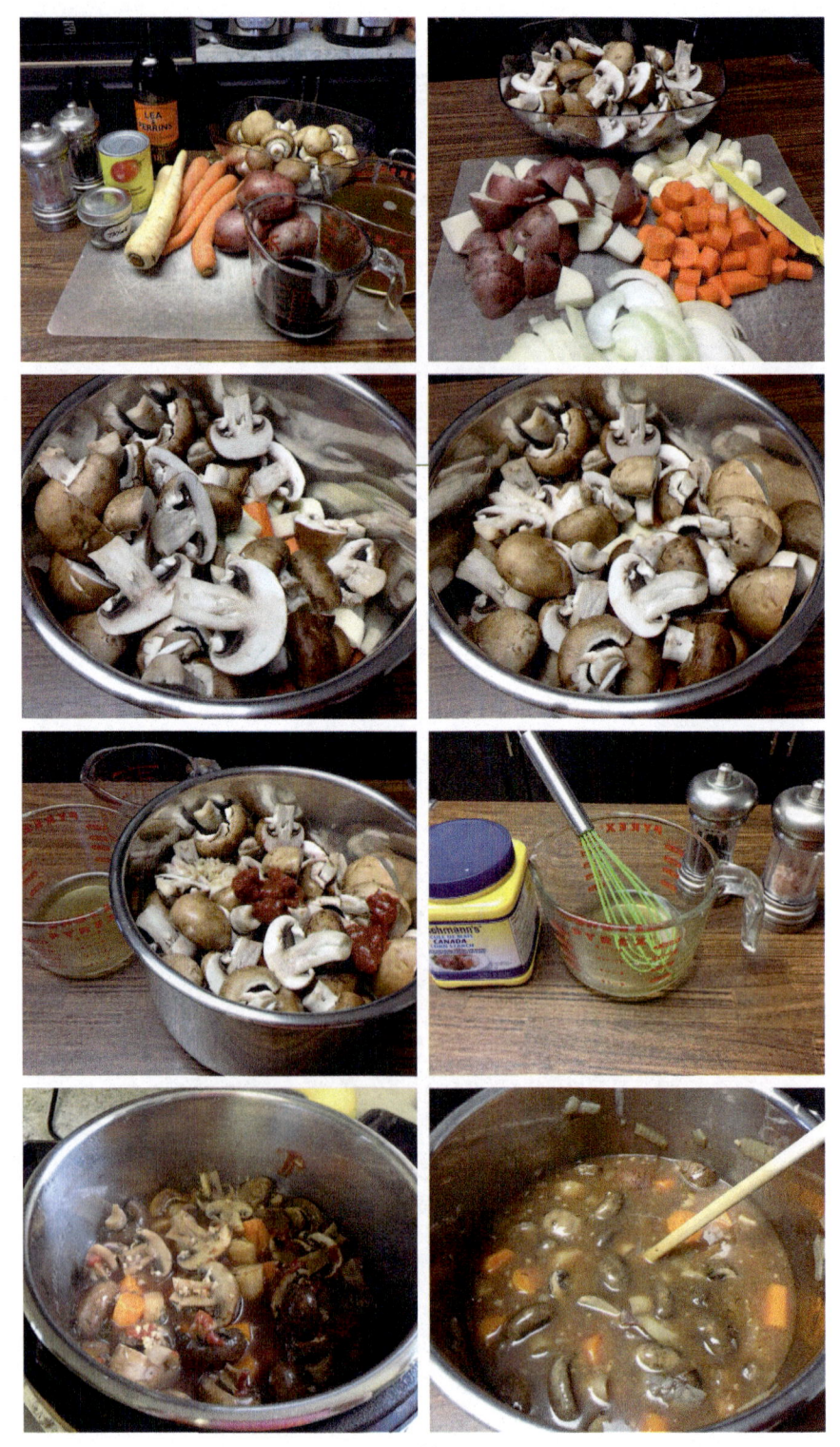

SIDE DISH RECIPES

RED CABBAGE AND APPLE

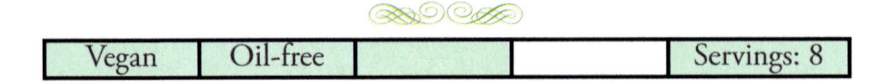

Vegan	Oil-free			Servings: 8

This low-calorie recipe can actually be either a side dish or a main dish. We like to pair it with vegan sausages. While the caraway seeds are optional, personally, we like the flavor it adds.

INGREDIENTS

3 tablespoons (45 ml) red wine vinegar or balsamic vinegar

½ cup (120 ml) vegetable broth or water

1 pound (450g) red cabbage, quartered, cored and thinly sliced

1 teaspoon (5 ml) sea salt

½ teaspoon (2.5 ml) caraway seeds

½ teaspoon (2.5 ml) black pepper, freshly ground

¼ teaspoon (2.5 ml) nutmeg, freshly grated

¼ teaspoon (2.5 ml) ground cinnamon

¼ teaspoon (2.5 ml) ground cloves

3 tablespoons (30g) brown sugar

1 medium yellow onion, halved and thinly sliced

2 apples, halved, cored and thinly sliced

2 cloves garlic, minced

DIRECTIONS

1. Add the vegetable broth (or water) and vinegar to the inner liner of your Instant Pot.
2. Tip: We've found that it's a good idea to take the inner liner out of your Instant Pot to the counter where you'll be working. You can

then add and layer all the ingredients and place the inner liner back in the Instant Pot before cooking. This lessens the danger of getting any of the ingredients into the lid channel.

3. Create a layer of cabbage (about ¼ of the head), sprinkle with about ¼ of the caraway seeds, spices and brown sugar. Then layer about ¼ of the thinly sliced onions, apples and garlic. Repeat until all of the ingredients are used up.
4. Return the inner liner to the Instant Pot.
5. Close and lock the lid ensuring the Pressure Valve is in the Sealing position.
6. Select the Steam function and set the cooking time for 3 minutes.
7. Once the cooking time is complete, do a Quick Release by carefully turning the Pressure Valve from Sealing to Venting.
8. Once all of the pressure has been released and the Float Valve has dropped, carefully remove the lid.
9. Stir well and serve immediately.

Nutritional Information per Serving:

Nutritional Information per Serving			
Servings	8		
Calories: 65		**Total fat:** 0.14g	
Calories from fat: 1 (1%)		Saturated: 0.05g	
Total Carbohydrates: 16.43g		Monounsaturated: 0.02g	
Dietary Fiber: 2.13g		Polyunsaturated: 0.07g	
Sugars: 11.98g		Trans fat: NA	
Cholesterol: --		**Sodium:** 367mg	
Protein 1.18g		**Potassium** 210mg	
Vitamin A:	680IU	**Vitamin C:** 35.24mg	**Calcium:** 39mg
Iron:	0.64mg	**Thiamin:** 0.05mg	**Niacin:** 0.30mg
Vitamin B6:	0.15mg	**Magnesium:** 13mg	**Folate:** 12µg

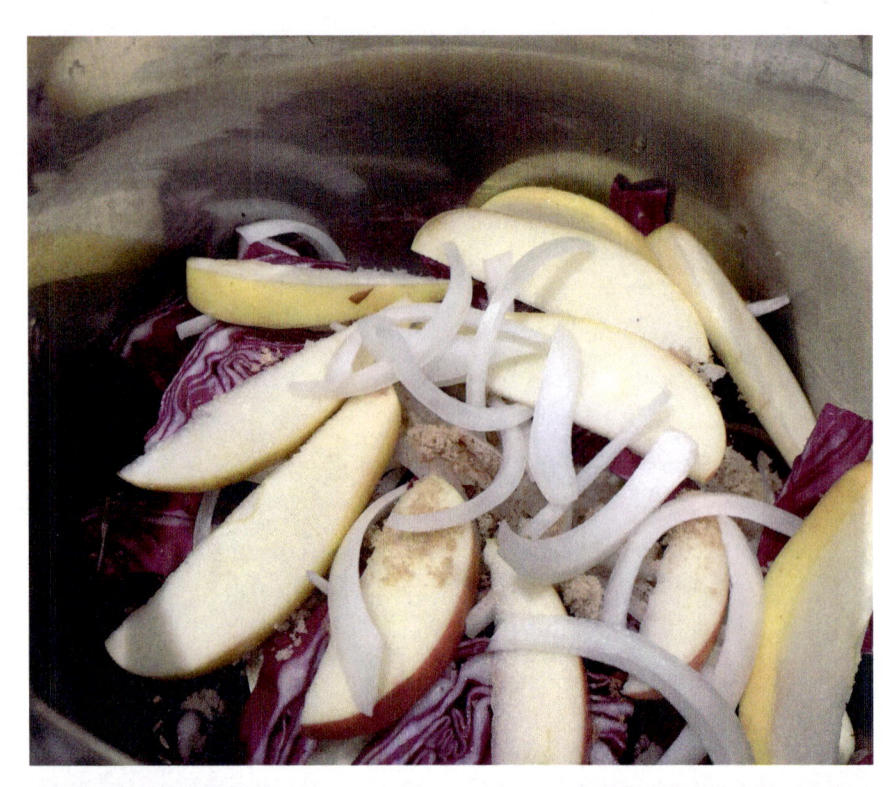

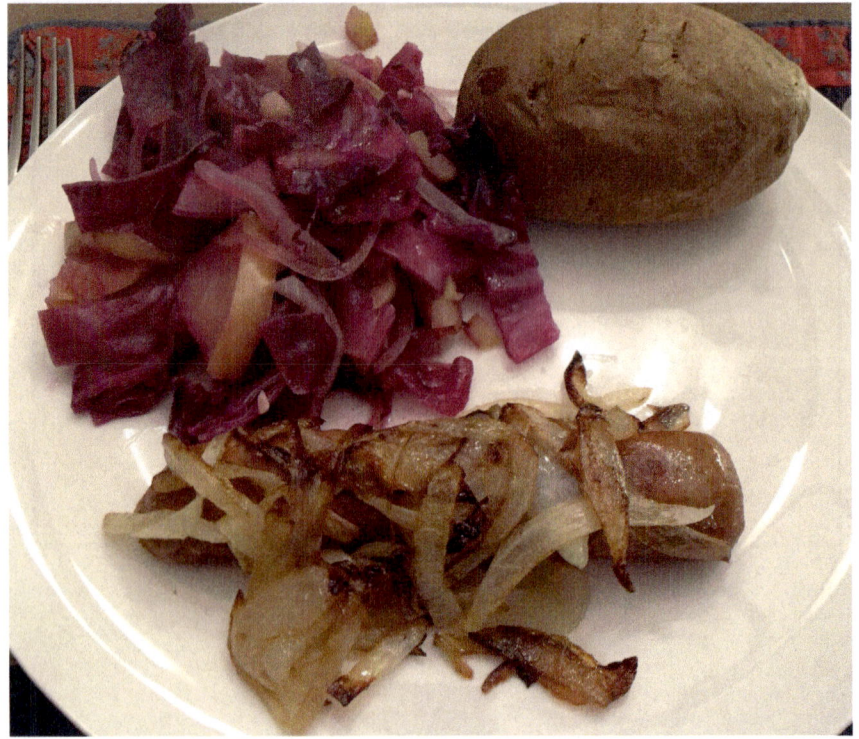

Cauliflower Tikka Masala

Vegan	Oil-free	WFPB		Servings: 8

INGREDIENTS

1 medium yellow onion, diced

3 cloves garlic, minced

1 inch (2.54 cm) piece ginger, peeled and minced

1 teaspoon (5 ml) fenugreek powder

2 teaspoons (10 ml) garam masala

1 teaspoon (5 ml) turmeric

½ teaspoon (2.5 ml) cumin

1 teaspoon (5 ml) chili powder

½ teaspoon (2.5 ml) sea salt

½ cup (120 ml) water

1 tablespoon (15 ml) maple syrup

1 head cauliflower, cut into florets

28 ounces (795g) diced tomatoes, canned

½ cup (120 ml) coconut milk

DIRECTIONS

1. Add all the ingredients, in the order given, with the exception of the coconut milk, to the inner liner of your Instant Pot. DO NOT STIR. (We don't stir this recipe because we don't want the tomatoes in contact with the bottom of the inner liner. This could cause a BURN notice.)
2. Close and lock the lid ensuring the Pressure Valve is in the Sealing position.

3. Select Pressure Cook/Manual mode and set the cooking time for 0 minutes. (No, that's not a mistake, you want to set the cooking time for ZERO minutes. If you set it for longer the cauliflower will overcook and you'll end up with mush.)
4. When cooking time is complete, immediately do a Quick Release (QR) by carefully turning the Pressure Valve from Sealing to Venting.
5. Once all of the pressure has been released, carefully remove the lid and remove the liner to a heatproof surface.
6. Add the coconut milk, stir gently and serve immediately.
7. You can freeze any leftovers, however, the cauliflower could become mushy when reheated.

Useful Information on total cooking time:

Time to come to pressure: approx. 15 minutes

Cooking time: 0 minutes

QR: time for pressure to release: approx. 1-2 minutes

Total Instant Pot time: approx. 16-17 minutes

Nutritional Information per Serving:

Nutritional Information per Serving	
Servings	8
Calories: 88	Total fat: 3.28g
Calories from fat: 29 (33%)	Saturated: 2.81g
Total Carbohydrates: 14.10g	Monounsaturated: 0.26g
Dietary Fiber: 3.49g	Polyunsaturated: 0.21g
Sugars: 7.18g	Trans fat: NA
Cholesterol: --	Sodium: 353mg
Protein 3.11g	Potassium 484mg
Vitamin A: 315IU	Vitamin C: 26.64mg	Calcium: 58mg
Iron: 2.68mg	Thiamin: 0.10mg	Niacin: 1.63mg
Vitamin B6: 0.26mg	Magnesium: 38mg	Folate: 36µg

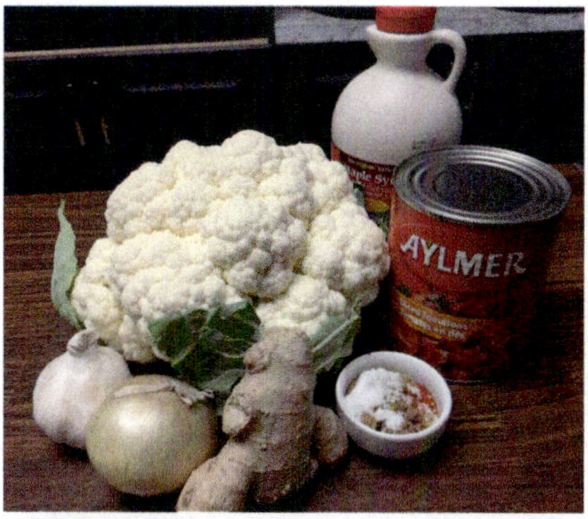
AYLMER
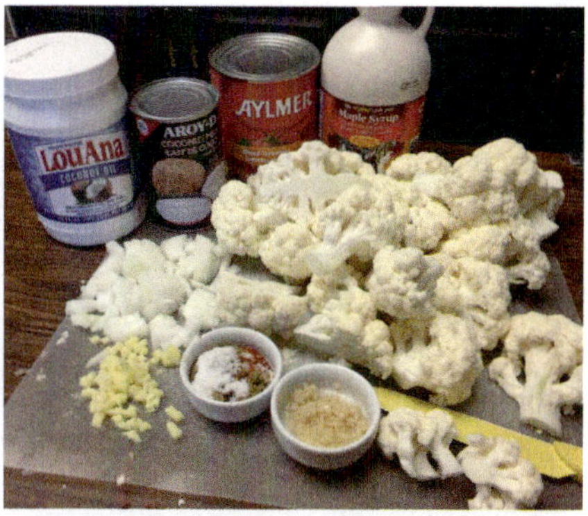
LouAna
AROY-D
AYLMER
Maple Syrup
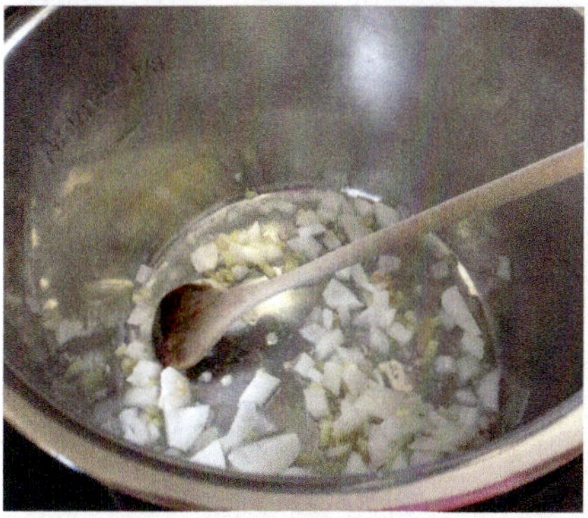
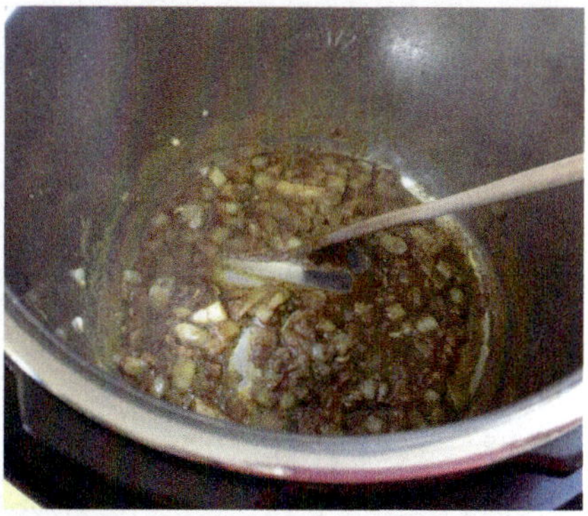
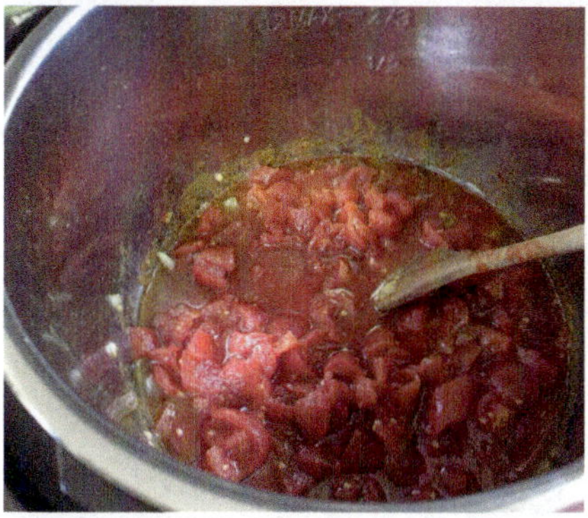
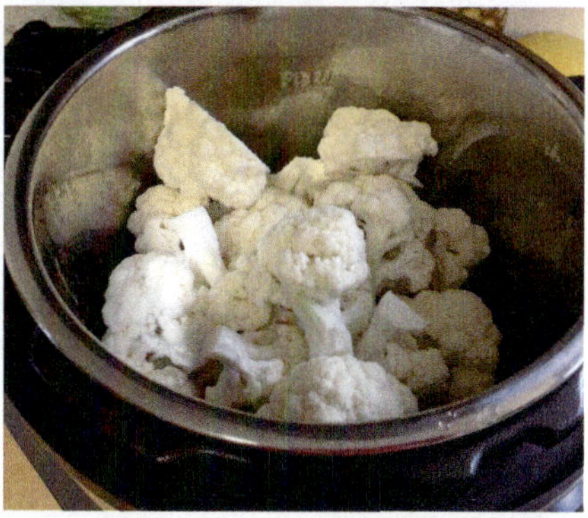
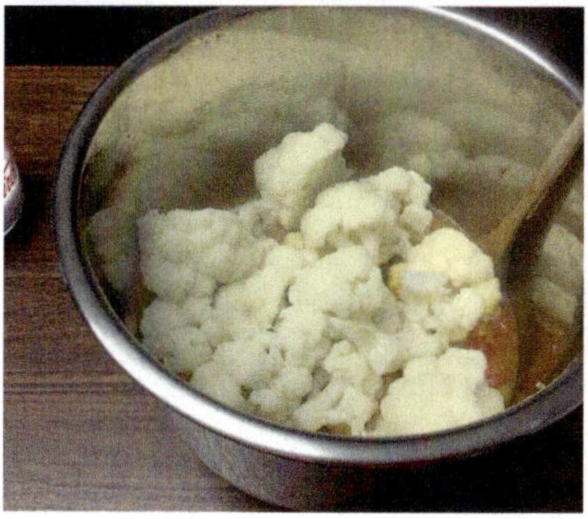
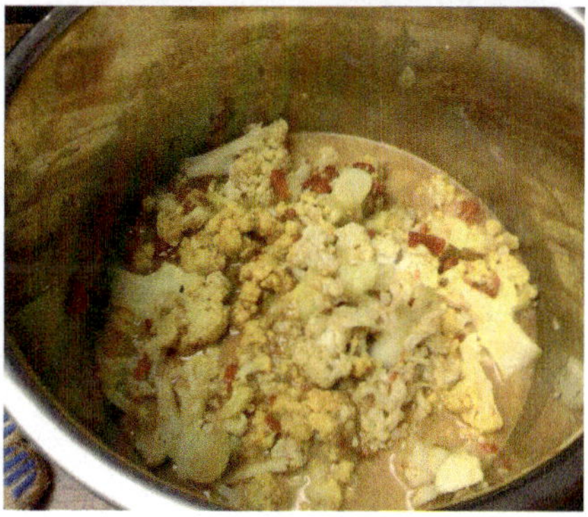

Brown Rice Risotto with Sugar Snap Peas

| Vegetarian | | | Servings: 6 |

We like to grow sugar snap peas in our garden every year and they go great in this brown rice risotto.

INGREDIENTS

1 teaspoon (5 ml) extra virgin olive oil

1 medium yellow onion, diced

1½ cups (375g) short grain brown rice

½ cup (120 ml) dry red or white wine

3½ cups (820 ml) vegetable broth, preferably homemade

½ teaspoon (2.5 ml) sea salt

½ teaspoon (2.5 ml) black pepper

1 cup (100g) Cremini mushrooms, diced

1½ cups (100g) sugar snap peas, cut larger ones in half

½ cup (75g) frozen green peas

¾ cup (75g) cheese, grated, cheddar or Parmesan (omit the cheese, or use vegan cheese, if you want the recipe to be vegan)

DIRECTIONS

1. Select Sauté mode on your Instant Pot and allow the inner liner to heat up.
2. Add the olive oil and allow it to heat up.
3. Add the diced onion and sauté for 2-3 minutes.
4. Add the rice and sauté for another 30 seconds to a minute.
5. Turn off Sauté mode.

6. Add the wine and the vegetable broth.
7. Stir well, using a wooden spoon to scrape any bits off the bottom of the pot.
8. Close and lock the lid ensuring the Pressure Valve is in the Sealing position.
9. Select Pressure Cook/Manual mode and set the cooking time for 30 minutes.
10. When cooking time is complete, allow a 5-minute Natural Pressure Release (NPR). Then release the rest of the pressure by carefully turning the Pressure Valve from Sealing to Venting.
11. Once all of the pressure has been released and the Float Valve has dropped, carefully remove the lid.
12. Add the diced mushrooms and the peas and stir well.
13. Add the cheese, if using, and stir well.
14. Leave the Instant Pot on Keep Warm to allow the mushrooms and the peas to heat through.
15. You can then serve immediately or leave it on Keep Warm until the rest of your meal is ready.

Useful Information on total cooking time:

Time to come to pressure: approx. 10 minutes

Cooking time: 30 minutes

NPR: 5 minutes

QR: time for pressure to release: approx. 2-3 minutes

Total Instant Pot time: approx. 47-48 minutes

Nutritional Information per Serving:

Nutritional Information per Serving		
Servings	6	
Calories: 290		**Total fat:** 4.50g
Calories from fat: 40 (13%)		Saturated: 2.04g
Total Carbohydrates: 48.06g		Monounsaturated: 1.73g
Dietary Fiber: 4.51g		Polyunsaturated: 0.73g
Sugars: 5.09g		Trans fat: NA
Cholesterol: 7mg	**Sodium:** 622mg	
Protein 10.56g	**Potassium** 365mg	
Vitamin A: 752IU	**Vitamin C:** 20.69mg	**Calcium:** 163mg
Iron: 1.78mg	**Thiamin:** 0.34mg	**Niacin:** 3.58mg
Vitamin B6: 0.37mg	**Magnesium:** 93mg	**Folate:** 50μg

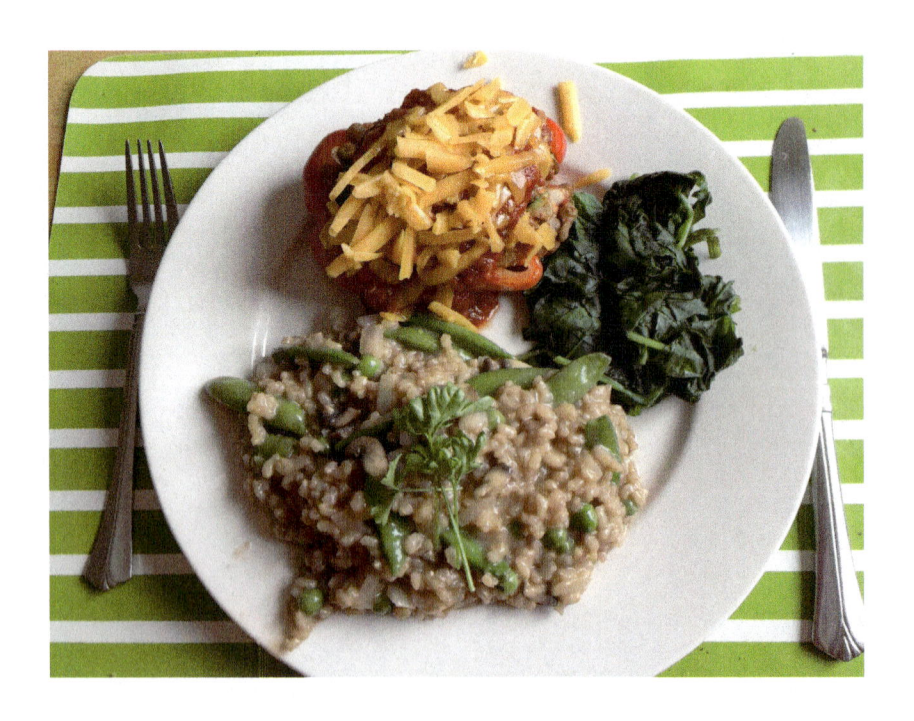

Easy, Pot-In-Pot, Brown Rice

| Vegan | Oil-free | WFPB | | Servings: 2 |

This is something we make all the time for just the two of us, so the measurements here are for two servings. For some this may seem like too much, for others, not enough. But this is what works for us. Feel free to adjust the recipe to suit your needs.

INGREDIENTS

⅔ cup (150g) brown rice, rinsed

1 cup (240 ml) water or vegetable broth

DIRECTIONS

1. Place one cup (240 ml) water in the inner liner of your Instant Pot and then place the trivet in the liner.

2. In a separate, oven-safe bowl/container, combine the brown rice and water (or vegetable broth) and give it a good stir.

3. Carefully place the bowl/container on the trivet, using a foil sling, if necessary. Note: There is no need to cover the bowl because it doesn't matter if a little extra water or steam gets into the rice.

4. Close and lock the lid of your Instant Pot, ensuring the Pressure Valve is in the Sealing position.

5. Select the Pressure Cook/Manual button and set the cooking time for 22 minutes.

6. Once cooking time is complete, allow AT LEAST a 10-minute NPR (Natural Pressure Release). Note: You can actually let the rice sit in the Instant Pot until the Float Valve drops on its own, if the rest of your meal isn't ready yet. And it can continue to stay on Keep Warm for a reasonable amount of time after that, too.

7. If you are releasing the pressure after the 10-minute NPR, do that by carefully turning the Pressure Valve from Sealing to Venting.
8. Once all the pressure has been released, and the Float Valve has dropped, carefully remove the lid.
9. Then, carefully remove the bowl from the inner liner either using the foil sling (if you used one) or with heatproof oven mitts, to a heatproof surface.
10. Fluff the rice with a fork and serve immediately.
11. As we make our rice fresh each time, we don't suggest refrigerating or freezing it. It's just so easy to make this way, there's no reason not to make it fresh each time.

Nutritional Information per Serving:

Nutritional Information per Serving		
Servings 2		
Calories: 229	**Total fat:** 1.55g	
Calories from fat: 13 (6%)	Saturated: 0.34g	
Total Carbohydrates: 48.24g	Monounsaturated: 0.61g	
Dietary Fiber: 2.15g	Polyunsaturated: 0.60g	
Sugars: --	Trans fat: NA	
Cholesterol: --	**Sodium:** 7mg	
Protein 4.75g	**Potassium** 169mg	
Vitamin A: --	**Vitamin C:** --	**Calcium:** 24mg
Iron: 1.14mg	**Thiamin:** 0.26mg	**Niacin:** 2.72mg
Vitamin B6: 0.32mg	**Magnesium:** 91mg	**Folate:** 12µg

79

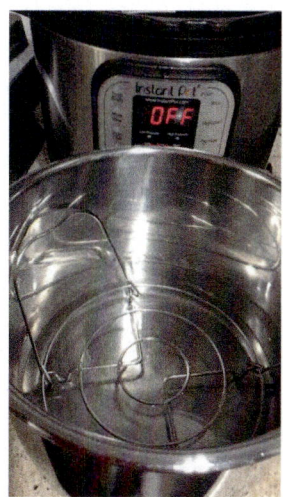

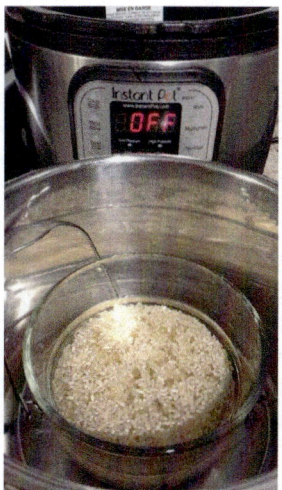

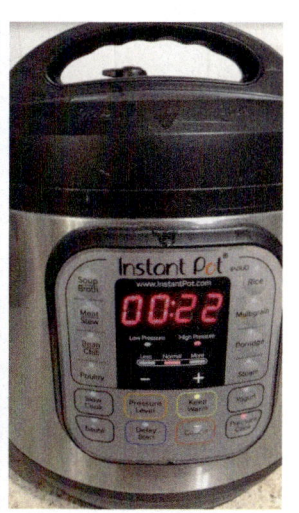

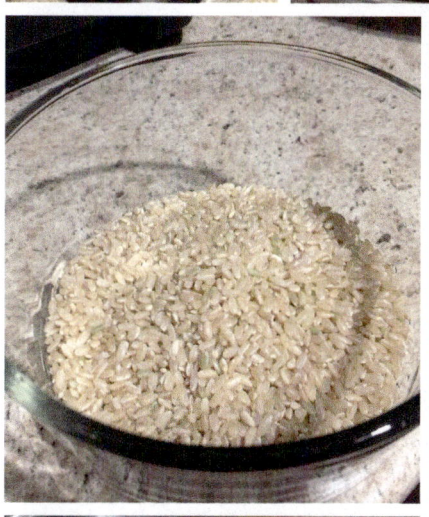

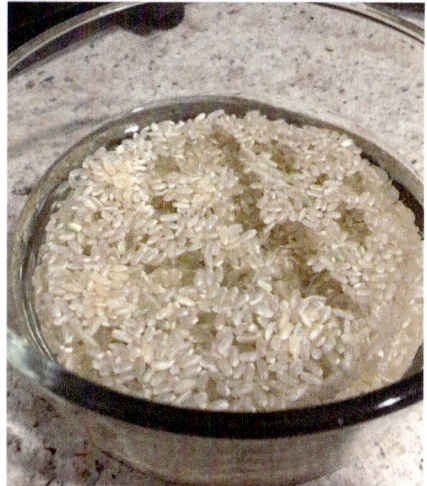

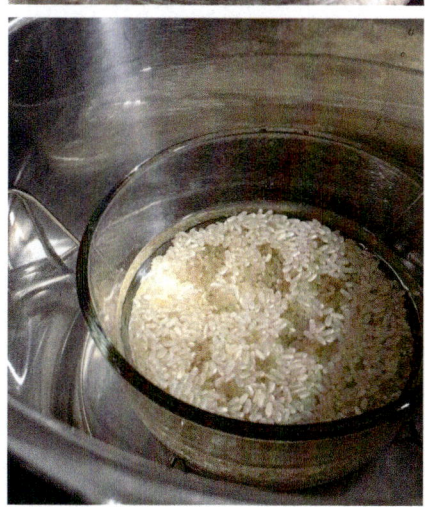

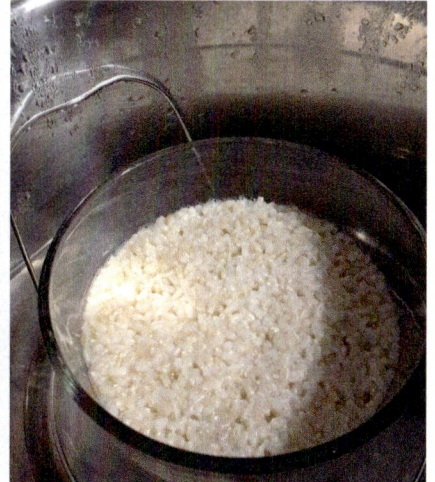

SOUP RECIPES

Asian Style Corn Soup

| Vegan | Oil-free | | | Servings: 4 |

INGREDIENTS

1½ cups (265g) corn kernels, fresh or frozen

10 ounces (295 ml) cream corn, canned

½ small red onion, diced

3 small carrots, chopped

2 cloves garlic, minced

1 small yellow onion, chopped

1 teaspoon (5 ml) sea salt

½ teaspoon (2.5 ml) black pepper, freshly ground

6 cups (1070 ml) vegetable broth

½ teaspoon (2.5 ml) Sriracha sauce OR any other Asian chili or chili-garlic sauce OR just use your favorite hot sauce to taste

SLURRY INGREDIENTS FOR THICKENING THE SOUP

1½ tablespoons (22.5 ml) all-purpose flour

1 tablespoon (15 ml) soy sauce

6 tablespoons (90 ml) water

DIRECTIONS

1. Add all the ingredients, with the exception of the Slurry Ingredients, to the inner liner of your Instant Pot.
2. Close and lock the lid ensuring the Pressure Valve is in the Sealing Position.

3. Select Soup/Broth Mode and set the cooking time for 2 minutes.
4. When cooking time is complete, allow a Natural Pressure Release for 10 minutes, then do a Quick Release (QR) by carefully turning the Pressure Valve from Sealing to Venting.
5. Once all of the pressure has been released, and the Float Valve has dropped, carefully remove the lid.
6. Press the Cancel button and then press the Sauté button.
7. Prepare the Slurry and slowly add it to the soup, stirring constantly.
8. Once the soup has thickened, press the Cancel button.
9. Carefully remove the inner liner to a heatproof surface and serve immediately or refrigerate or freeze for later use.
10. Note: We actually did this recipe in an 8 Quart Instant Pot but the timing will be the same for a 6 Quart.

Nutritional Information per Serving:

Nutritional Information per Serving	
Servings 4	
Calories: 168	**Total fat:** 1.05g
Calories from fat: 9 (5%)	Saturated: 0.25g
Total Carbohydrates: 39.79g	Monounsaturated: 0.33g
Dietary Fiber: 3.89g	Polyunsaturated: 0.47g
Sugars: 12.61g	Trans fat: NA
Cholesterol: --	**Sodium:** 1848mg
Protein 4.69g	**Potassium** 456mg
Vitamin A: 7119IU	**Vitamin C:** 12.92mg	**Calcium:** 34mg
Iron: 0.94mg	**Thiamin:** 0.15mg	**Niacin:** 2.26mg
Vitamin B6: 0.24mg	**Magnesium:** 44mg	**Folate:** 76µg

CREAMY TOMATO SOUP

| Vegetarian* | Oil-free | | | Servings: 6 |

Note. Vegan (with a single substitution)

Made with fresh Roma (plum tomatoes) this recipe is also oil-free and can be vegan with a simple substitution as noted in the list of ingredients.

INGREDIENTS

1 cup (240 ml) vegetable broth, preferably homemade

3½ pounds (2.6 Kg) Roma (plum) tomatoes, diced

½ medium yellow onion, diced

1 tablespoon (15 ml) honey, (sub sugar for vegan)

3 cloves garlic, minced

1 tablespoon (15 ml) basil

1 teaspoon (5 ml) sea salt

2 tablespoons (30 ml) Poblano lime sauce, or spicy sauce of your choice, optional

½ cup (120 ml) oat milk or plant-based milk of your choice

DIRECTIONS

1. Add all the ingredients, with the exception of the plant-based milk, in the order given, to the inner liner of your Instant Pot.
2. DO NOT STIR. (Sometimes tomatoes can result in the dreaded BURN notice, so we like to make sure they have the cushion of the vegetable broth while cooking.)
3. Close and lock the lid ensuring the Pressure Valve is in the Sealing position.

4. Select the Soup/Broth mode and set the cooking time for 7 minutes.
5. When cooking time is complete allow a 10-minute Natural Pressure Release followed by a Quick Release (QR) by carefully turning the Pressure Valve from Sealing to Venting.
6. Once the rest of the pressure has been released, and the Float Valve has dropped, carefully remove the lid.
7. Using a blender (we used a VitaMix), purée the soup in batches until smooth.
8. Add the plant-based milk and stir well.
9. Serve immediately or refrigerate or freeze for later use.

Nutritional Information Per Serving

Nutritional Information per Serving		
Servings 6		
Calories: 80	**Total fat:** 0.58g	
Calories from fat: 5 (6%)	Saturated: 0.06g	
Total Carbohydrates: 18.02g	Monounsaturated: 0.09g	
Dietary Fiber: 3.51g	Polyunsaturated: 0.22g	
Sugars: 13.04g	Trans fat: NA	
Cholesterol: --	**Sodium:** 563mg	
Protein 2.68g	**Potassium** 662mg	
Vitamin A: 2323IU	**Vitamin C:** 37.53mg	**Calcium:** 33mg
Iron: 0.83mg	**Thiamin:** 0.09mg	**Niacin:** 1.62mg
Vitamin B6: 0.25mg	**Magnesium:** 31mg	**Folate:** 41μg

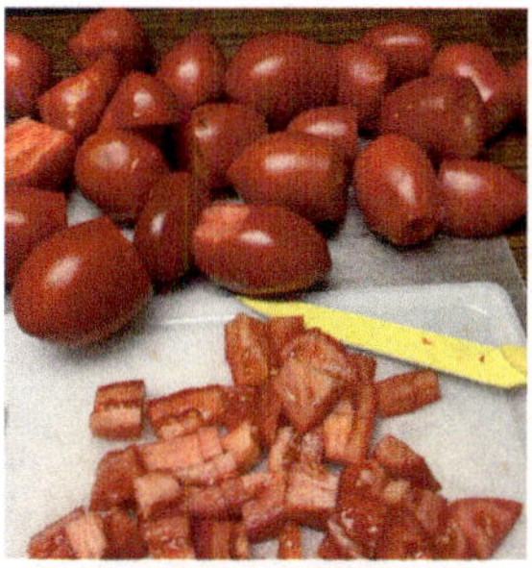
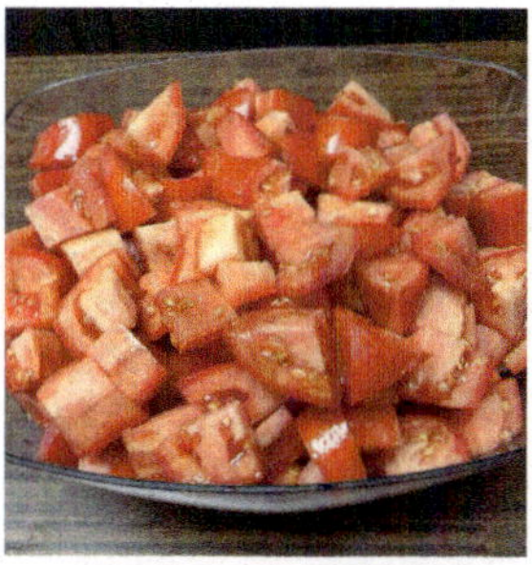
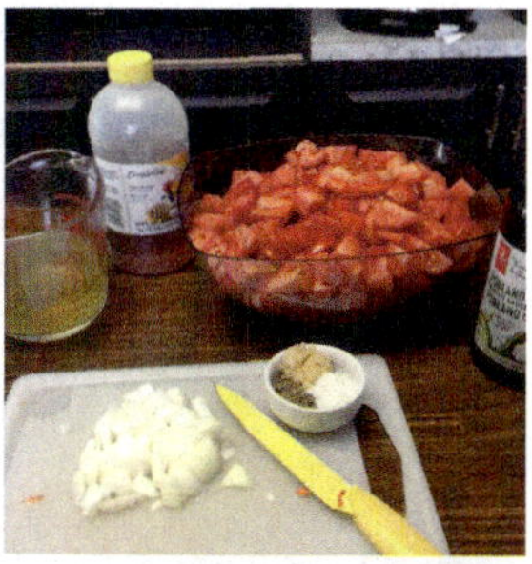
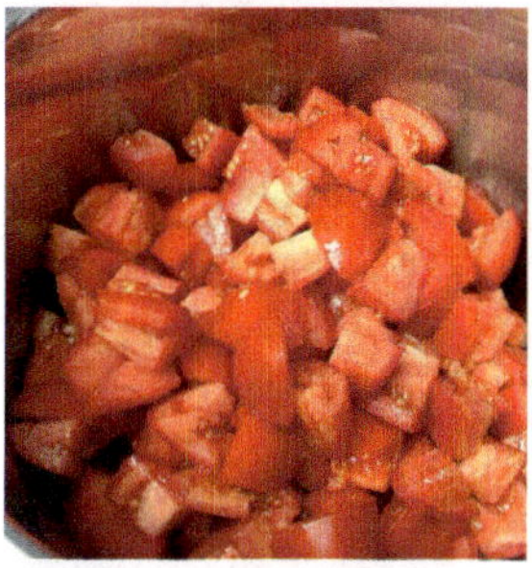
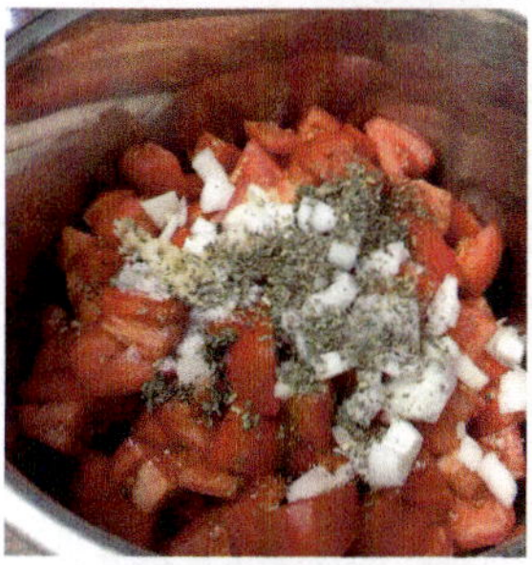
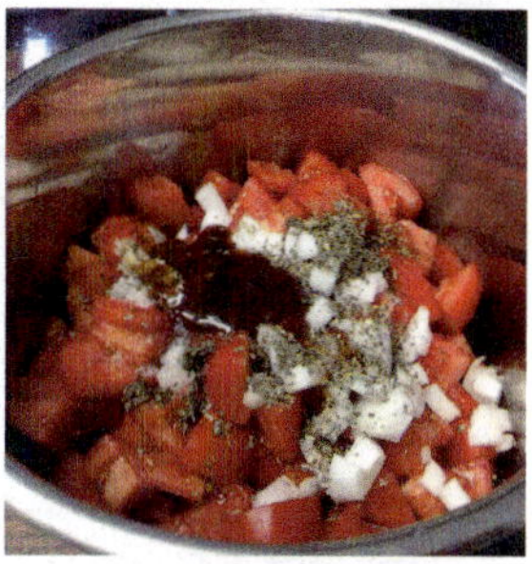
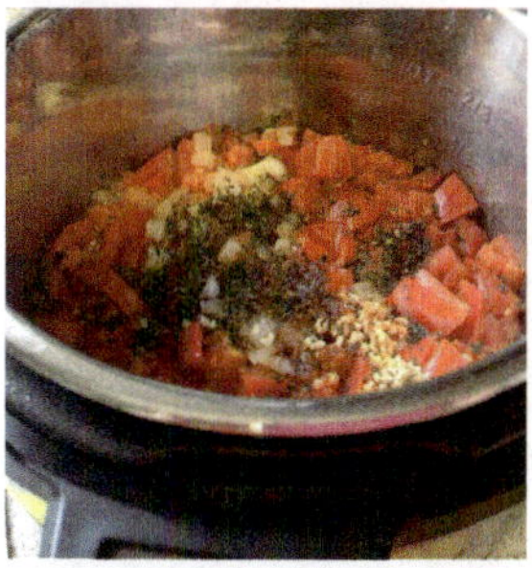
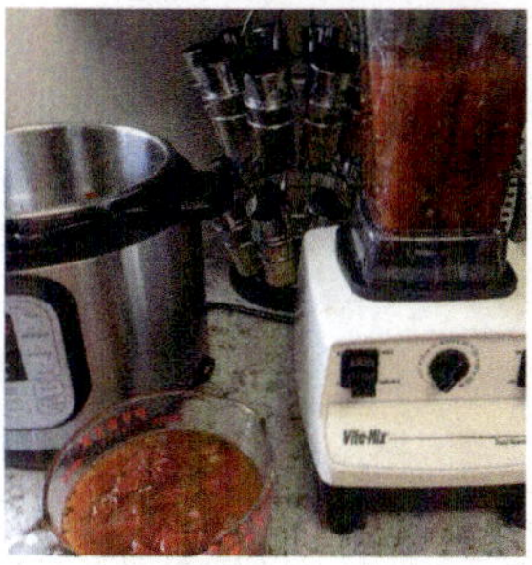
Vita-Mix
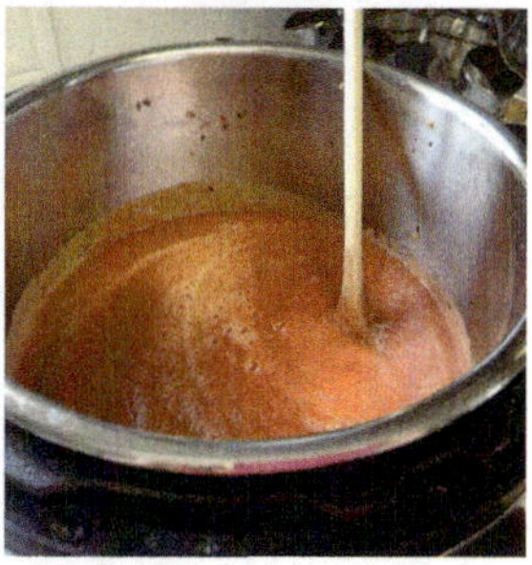
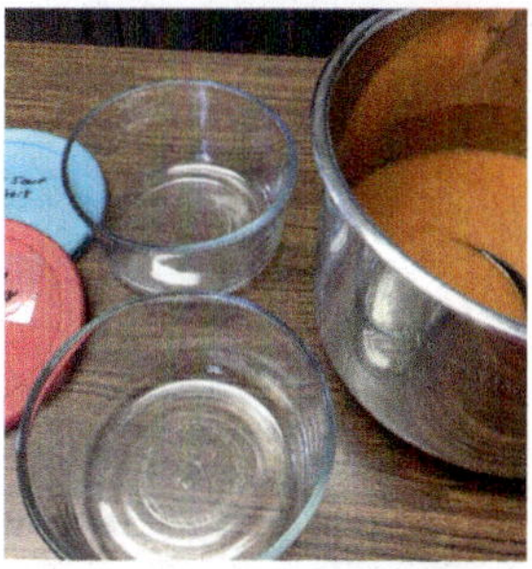
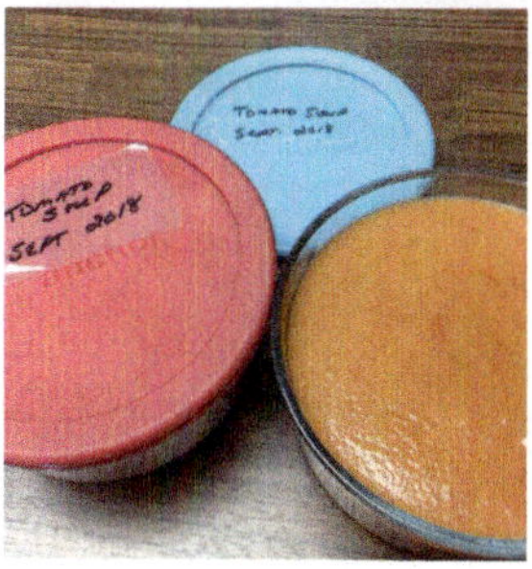
TOMATO SOUP SEPT 2018
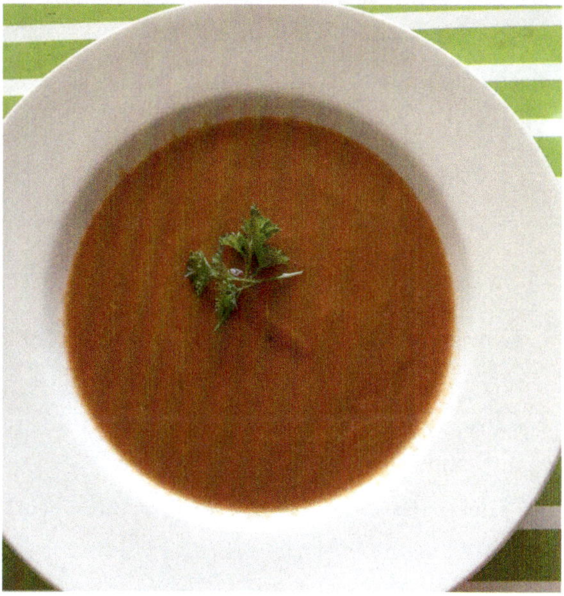

Detox Vegetable and Red Lentil Soup

Vegan	Oil-free	WFPB		Servings: 8

INGREDIENTS

6 cups (1.4 L) vegetable broth, preferably homemade

1 cup (200g) red lentils

1 large yellow onion, diced

4 cloves garlic, minced

1 inch piece (2.54 cm) ginger, minced

4 stalks celery, sliced

2 cups (175g) broccoli, florets, chopped

1 cup (110g) cauliflower, florets, chopped

2 teaspoons (10 ml) turmeric

2 teaspoons (10 ml) chili powder

1½ teaspoons (7.5 ml) sea salt

1 teaspoon (5 ml) black pepper, freshly ground

28 ounces (795g) canned tomatoes, diced

DIRECTIONS

1. Combine all the ingredients, in the order given, in the inner liner of your Instant Pot. DO NOT STIR.
2. Close and lock the lid ensuring the Pressure Valve is in the Sealing position.
3. Select the Soup/Broth mode and set the cooking time for 5 minutes.

4. When cooking time is complete, allow a 10-minute Natural Pressure Release (NPR). This allows the contents to settle down before releasing the rest of the pressure.
5. After the 10-minute NPR, release the rest of the pressure by carefully turning the Pressure Valve from Sealing to Venting.
6. Once all of the pressure has been released, and the Float Valve has dropped, carefully remove the lid.
7. Stir well and serve immediately. Or, refrigerate or freeze for later use.

Useful Information on total cooking time:

Time to come to pressure: approx. 28 minutes

Cooking time: 5 minutes

NPR: 10 minutes

QR: time for pressure to release: approx. 2-3 minutes

Total Instant Pot time: approx. 45-46 minutes

Note: We used an 8-quart Instant Pot Duo for this recipe but it should work equally as well in a 6 quart.

Nutritional Information per Serving:

Nutritional Information per Serving		
Servings 8		
Calories: 141	**Total fat:** 0.63g	
Calories from fat: 5 (4%)	Saturated: 0.16g	
Total Carbohydrates: 27.76g	Monounsaturated: 0.13g	
Dietary Fiber: 6.74g	Polyunsaturated: 0.33g	
Sugars: 6.49g	Trans fat: NA	
Cholesterol: --	**Sodium:** 1021mg	
Protein 8.37g	**Potassium** 620mg	
Vitamin A: 1276IU	**Vitamin C:** 43.18mg	**Calcium:** 79mg
Iron: 3.17mg	**Thiamin:** 0.82mg	**Niacin:** 1.83mg
Vitamin B6: 0.38mg	**Magnesium:** 37mg	**Folate:** 159µg

88

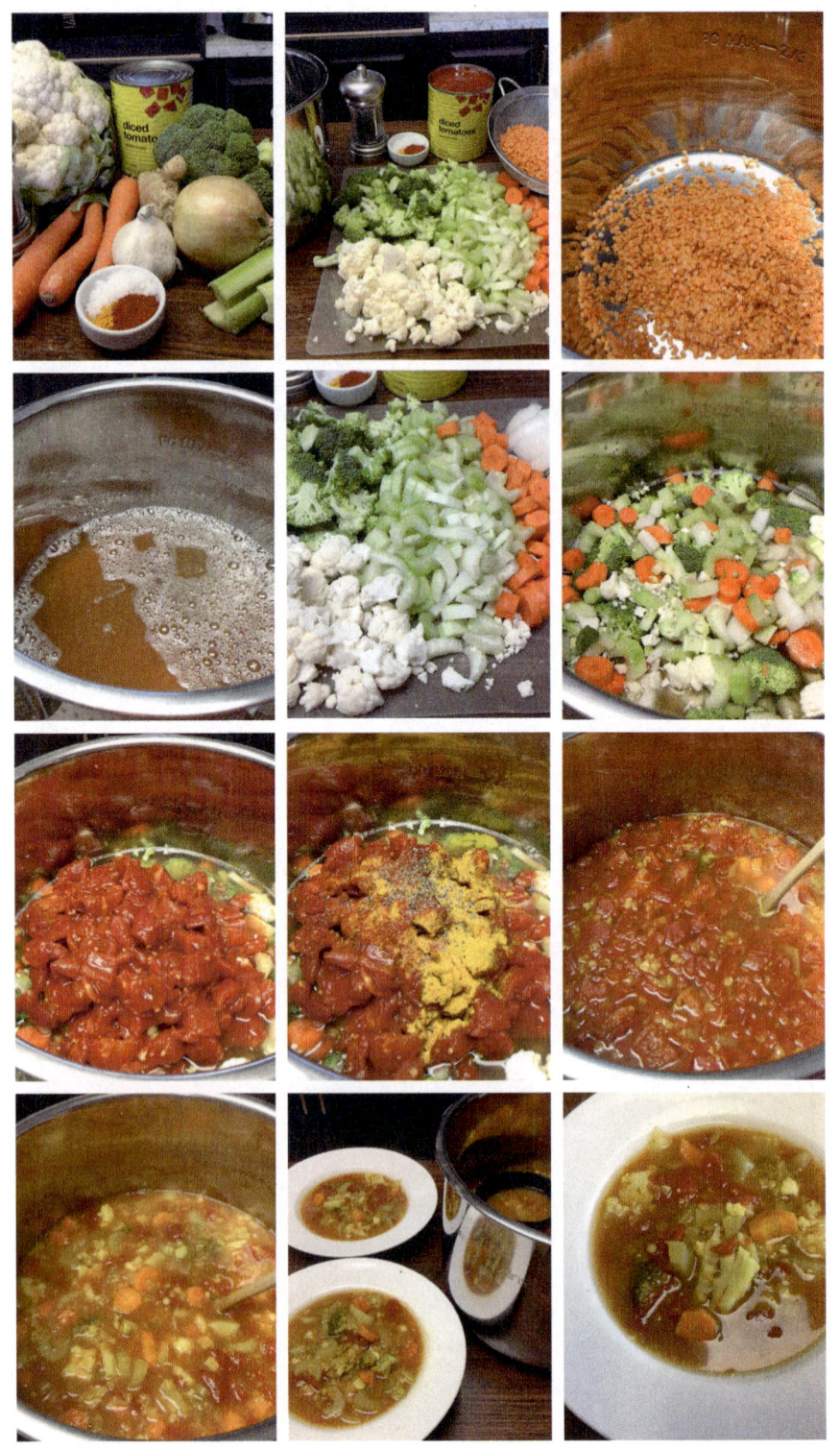

Lentil and Yam Soup

| Vegan | Oil-free | WFPB | | Servings: 6 |

INGREDIENTS

1 medium yellow onion, chopped

1 large celery stalk, diced

4 cloves garlic, minced

1 teaspoon (5 ml) ground cumin

1 teaspoon (5 ml) paprika

1 teaspoon (5 ml) salt

1 teaspoon (5 ml) black pepper

½ teaspoon (2.5 ml) red pepper flakes

1 cup (200g) green lentils

16 ounces (454g) yams (sweet potatoes), peeled and large dice

3½ cups (820 ml) vegetable broth

1 cup (240 ml) water

14 ounces (400g) diced tomatoes, canned, with juice

4 ounces (114g) baby spinach, well washed and dried (we like to use a salad spinner)

DIRECTIONS

1. Add all the ingredients to the inner liner of your Instant Pot, with the exception of the baby spinach, and stir.
2. Close and lock the lid ensuring the Pressure Valve is in the Sealing position.
3. Select the Soup/Broth mode and set the cooking time for 12 minutes.

4. Once cooking time is complete, allow a 10-minute NPR (Natural Pressure Release) and then release the rest of the pressure by carefully turning the Pressure Valve from Sealing to Venting.
5. When all of the pressure has been released and the Float Valve has dropped, carefully remove the lid.
6. Add the spinach and stir until everything is well combined and the spinach has wilted.
7. Carefully remove the inner liner to a heatproof surface.
8. Serve immediately or refrigerate or freeze for later use.

Useful Information on total cooking time:

Time to come to pressure: approx. 25 minutes (Note: we used semi-frozen vegetable broth in this recipe.)

Cooking time: 12 minutes

NPR: 10 minutes

QR: time for pressure to release: approx. 3 minutes

Total Instant Pot time: 50 minutes

Nutritional Information per Serving:

Nutritional Information per Serving		
Servings 6		
Calories: 249	**Total fat:** 0.70g	
Calories from fat: 6 (2%)	Saturated: 0.15g	
Total Carbohydrates: 51.99g	Monounsaturated: 0.16g	
Dietary Fiber: 9.03g	Polyunsaturated: 0.39g	
Sugars: 6.19g	Trans fat: NA	
Cholesterol: --	**Sodium:** 866mg	
Protein 11.24g	**Potassium** 1217mg	
Vitamin A: 2628IU	**Vitamin C:** 28.22mg	**Calcium:** 84mg
Iron: 4.32mg	**Thiamin:** 0.44mg	**Niacin:** 2.33mg
Vitamin B6: 0.60mg	**Magnesium:** 65mg	**Folate:** 222µg

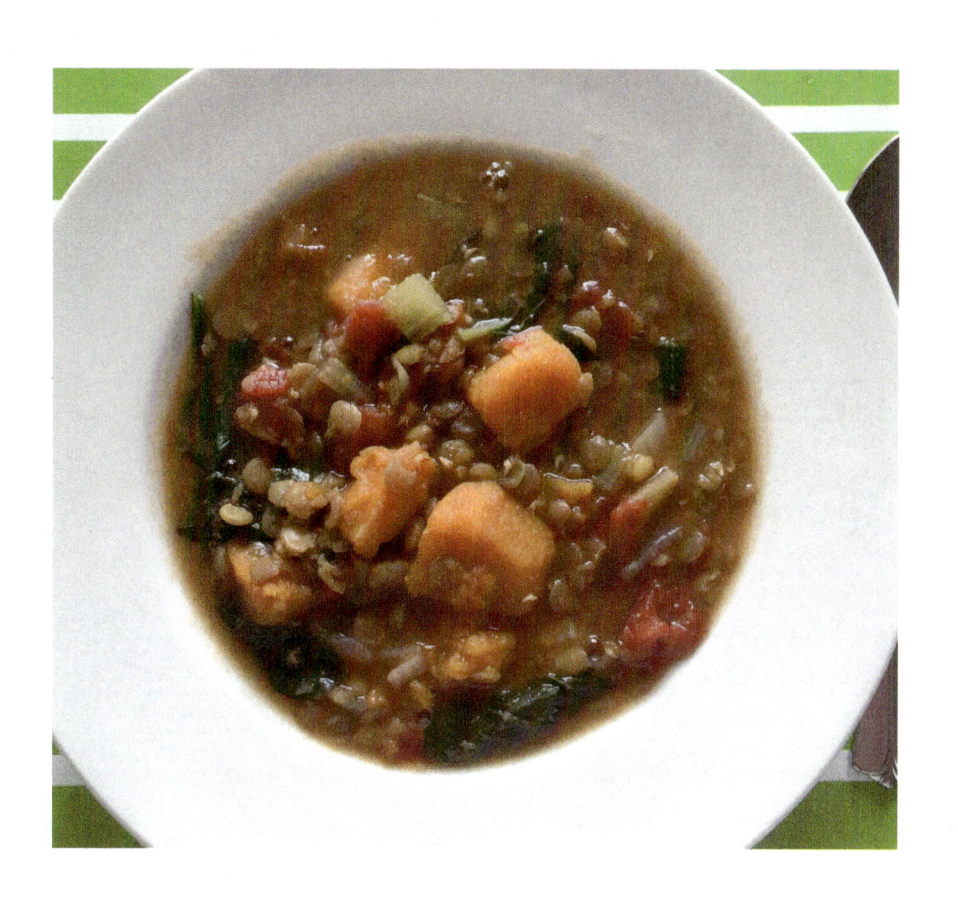

Italian Inspired Pasta Soup

| Vegan | Oil-free | WFPB | | Servings: 8 |

Not minestrone but still tasty and filling.

INGREDIENTS

- 3 cups (700 ml) vegetable broth, preferably homemade
- 5 ounces (142g) pasta, your choice
- 1 small red onion, chopped
- 4 cloves garlic, minced
- 1 medium carrot, chopped
- ½ medium green bell pepper, chopped
- 1 small zucchini, chopped
- 1½ cups (255g) kidney beans, cooked
- 1½ cups (350 ml) crushed tomatoes
- 2 tablespoons (30 ml) tomato paste
- 1 large tomato, diced
- 1 cup (100g) baby spinach, packed, optional

DIRECTIONS

1. Add all ingredients, except the spinach, to the inner liner of your Instant Pot in the order given, making sure the pasta is covered by broth so it will cook properly. DO NOT STIR
2. Close and lock the lid, ensuring that the Pressure Valve is in the Sealing position.
3. Select the Pressure Cook/Manual mode and set the cooking time for 3 minutes.

4. Once the cooking time is complete, allow a 10-minute Natural Pressure Release.
5. Then release the rest of the pressure by carefully turning the Pressure Valve from Sealing to Venting.
6. When all of the pressure has been released, and the Float Valve has dropped, carefully remove the lid.
7. Add the spinach and stir well until all the spinach has wilted and all the ingredients are well combined.
8. Serve immediately or refrigerate or freeze for later use.

Nutritional Information per Serving:

Nutritional Information per Serving	
Servings 8	
Calories: 157	**Total fat:** 0.78g
Calories from fat: 7 (4%)	Saturated: 0.17g
Total Carbohydrates: 32.09g	Monounsaturated: 0.26g
Dietary Fiber: 5.24g	Polyunsaturated: 0.35g
Sugars: 8.24g	Trans fat: NA
Cholesterol: --	**Sodium:** 740mg
Protein 6.86g	**Potassium** 542mg
Vitamin A: 2229IU	**Vitamin C:** 21.36mg	**Calcium:** 71mg
Iron: 2.53mg	**Thiamin:** 0.29mg	**Niacin:** 2.58mg
Vitamin B6: 0.29mg	**Magnesium:** 48mg	**Folate:** 92µg

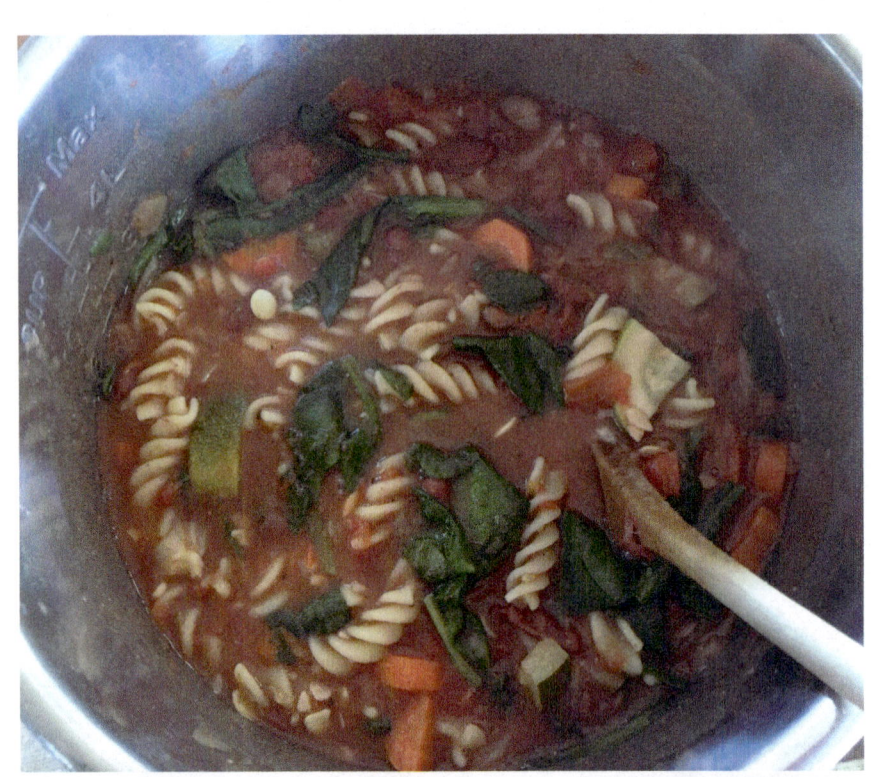

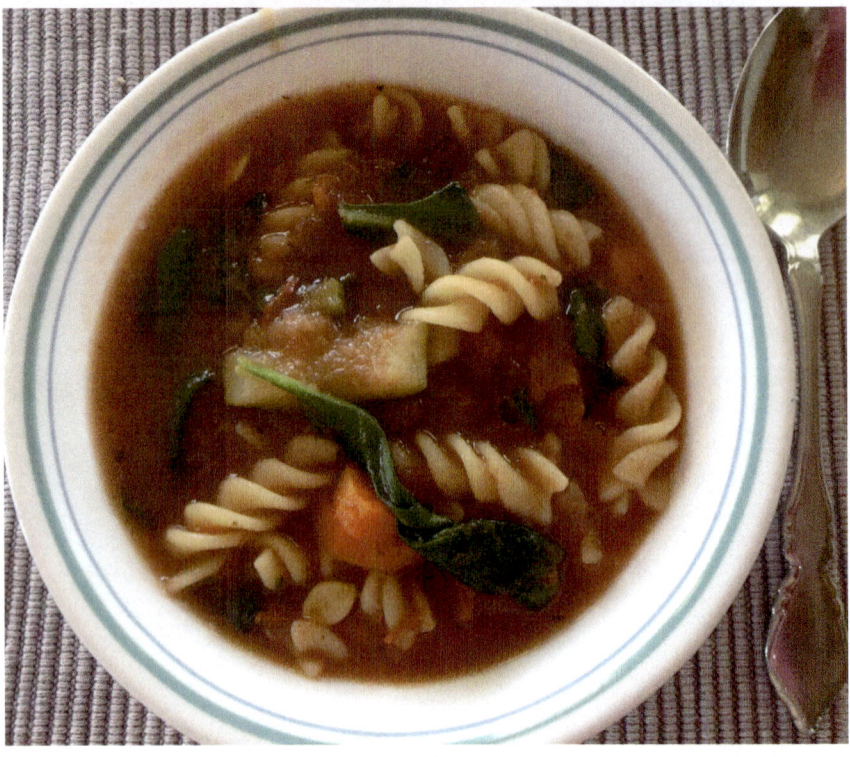

Black Bean Soup

Vegan	Oil-free	WFPB		Servings: 10

Super low calorie and tasty soup. At only 91 calories per serving, feel free to have a second helping!

INGREDIENTS

16 ounces (454g) black beans, dried

4 cups (950 ml) vegetable broth, preferably homemade

1 cup (240 ml) water

1 medium yellow onion, chopped

1 large bell pepper, chopped

3 stalks celery, chopped

1 tablespoon (15 ml) paprika

1 teaspoon (5 ml) hot sauce

1 tablespoon (15 ml) cumin

28 ounces (795 ml) canned tomatoes, whole

DIRECTIONS

1. Place all of the ingredients in the inner liner of your Instant Pot in the order given. DO NOT STIR (You don't want to stir this in case you get the tomatoes on the bottom, which could cause a BURN notice.)
2. Close and lock the lid ensuring the Pressure Valve is in the Sealing position.
3. Select the Bean/Chili button and set the cooking time for 22 minutes.

4. Once cooking time is complete, allow a Full NPR (Natural Pressure Release). That means, to just allow the pressure to release until the Float Valve drops on its own. That can take about 40-50 minutes.
5. When the Float Valve has dropped, carefully remove the lid and give the soup a good stir.
6. Serve immediately or refrigerate or freeze for later use.

Useful Information on total cooking time:

Time to come to pressure: approx. 20 minutes

(note: for this recipe we actually used frozen broth so, if you're using room temperature broth, it may not take as long to come to pressure.)

Cooking time: 22 minutes

Full NPR: approx. 40-50 minutes

Total Instant Pot time: approx. 62-72 minutes

Nutritional Information per Serving:

Nutritional Information per Serving	
Servings 10	
Calories: 91	**Total fat:** 0.56g
Calories from fat: 5 (5%)	Saturated: 0.13g
Total Carbohydrates: 17.71g	Monounsaturated: 0.15g
Dietary Fiber: 6.53g	Polyunsaturated: 0.28g
Sugars: 4.02g	Trans fat: NA
Cholesterol: --	**Sodium:** 439mg
Protein 5.25g	**Potassium** 433mg
Vitamin A: 1023IU	**Vitamin C:** 24.67mg	**Calcium:** 57mg
Iron: 2.07mg	**Thiamin:** 0.58mg	**Niacin:** 1.04mg
Vitamin B6: 0.20mg	**Magnesium:** 47mg	**Folate:** 84µg

Quick Potato Corn Chowder

| Vegan | Oil-free | | | Servings: 8 |

For some reason we had several cans of creamed corn in our pantry. Neither one of us likes creamed corn as a separate vegetable, so we're not quite sure why we had these. However, it gave us inspiration for a quick, tasty soup and a way to use up some of the cans. Here's what we did.

INGREDIENTS

4 cloves garlic, chopped

2 small yellow onions, chopped

6 medium size potatoes, large dice

2 teaspoons (10 ml) sea salt or Himalayan pink salt

1 teaspoon (5 ml) black pepper, freshly ground

1 teaspoon (5 ml) dried thyme

1 cup (240 ml) water

2 cups (480 ml) vegetable broth (preferably homemade)

---

1 cup (240 ml) cashew milk (or plant-based milk of your choice)

1½ tablespoons (22.5 ml) cornstarch

14-ounce (398 ml) canned creamed corn

1-2 tablespoons (15-30 ml) fresh parsley, chopped

DIRECTIONS

1. Add the first eight ingredients to the inner pot of your Instant Pot. Stir well.

2. Close and lock the lid ensuring that the Pressure Valve is in the Sealing position.
3. Select the Soup/Broth button and set cooking time for 8 minutes.
4. When cooking time is complete, allow a Natural Pressure Release for 4-5 minutes, then manually release the rest of the pressure by carefully turning the Pressure Valve from Sealing to Venting.
5. When the pressure has been completely released and the Float Valve has dropped, open and remove the lid and turn the Instant Pot off.
6. Now, select Sauté mode. This is so you can thicken the soup.
7. Whisk together the cashew milk and cornstarch. When the cornstarch is well dissolved in the cashew milk, pour it into the soup while stirring.
8. Add the can of creamed corn and stir.
9. Add the fresh parsley and stir.
10. Add more salt and pepper, to taste, if desired.
11. When the soup has reached the desired consistency, turn off your Instant Pot.
12. Serve immediately or refrigerate or freeze for later use.

Nutritional Information Per Serving:

Nutritional Information per Serving	
Servings 8	
Calories: 180	**Total fat:** 0.56g
Calories from fat: 5 (2%)	Saturated: 0.07g
Total Carbohydrates: 41.09g	Monounsaturated: 0.06g
Dietary Fiber: 3.26g	Polyunsaturated: 0.11g
Sugars: 3.51g	Trans fat: NA
Cholesterol: --	**Sodium:** 852mg
Protein 4.48g	**Potassium** 788mg
Vitamin A: 1186IU	**Vitamin C:** 28.13mg	**Calcium:** 49mg
Iron: 2.47mg	**Thiamin:** 0.15mg	**Niacin:** 1.97mg
Vitamin B6: 0.60mg	**Magnesium:** 48mg	**Folate:** 50µg

French Onion Soup

| Vegetarian | | | Servings: 8 |

This is amazingly easy to make and just as easy to dress up a bit with some toasted bread (or croutons) and some shredded cheese. It works well with a salad for lunch or as a first course for dinner.

INGREDIENTS

1 tablespoon (15 ml) extra virgin olive oil

1 tablespoon (15 ml) butter

1½ pounds (680g) onions (we used yellow onions from our garden)

4 cloves garlic, minced

1 cup (250 ml) dry red wine

4 cups (950 ml) vegetable broth

1 teaspoon (5 ml) dried thyme

1 teaspoon (5 ml) vegan Worcestershire sauce

1 bay leaf

1 teaspoon (5 ml) sea salt or Himalayan pink salt

1 teaspoon (5 ml) black pepper, freshly ground

Slices of French bread, toasted (or croutons)

Grated cheese of your choice (use vegan cheese, if desired)

DIRECTIONS

1. Cut the onions in half, lengthwise, then slice. Set aside.
2. Select Sauté mode on your Instant Pot and add the butter and olive oil. Heat until it begins to sizzle and bubble.
3. Add the onions and garlic. Stir frequently until the onions become translucent and there's a bit sticking to the bottom of the pan - about 10-12 minutes. The onions still need to be slightly firm, not mushy.
4. Add the red wine and stir to deglaze the pan.
5. Add the broth, Worcestershire sauce, thyme, bay leaf, salt and pepper. Stir.
6. Turn off Sauté mode.
7. Close and lock the lid ensuring the Pressure Valve is in the Sealing position.
8. Select Soup/Broth button and set cooking time for 8 minutes.
9. When cooking time is complete, do a Quick Release by carefully turning the Pressure Valve from Sealing to Venting.
10. Once all the pressure has been released, and the Float Valve has dropped, carefully remove the lid.
11. Carefully remove the inner liner to a heatproof surface and give the onion soup a good stir.
12. Ladle the soup into ovenproof, individual serving bowls and top with the toasted French bread or croutons and grated cheese.
13. Place under the broiler for a few minutes until the cheese starts to bubble and brown.
14. Tip: Place the bowls on a baking sheet before placing them under the broiler to make it easier to get them in and out of the oven.

Nutritional Information per Serving
(Not including the French bread/croutons or grated cheese.)

Nutritional Information per Serving		
Servings 8		
Calories: 186	**Total fat:** 3.19g	
Calories from fat: 28 (15%)	Saturated: 1.28g	
Total Carbohydrates: 32.39g	Monounsaturated: 1.64g	
Dietary Fiber: 5.49g	Polyunsaturated: 0.27g	
Sugars: 14.50g	Trans fat: NA	
Cholesterol: 3mg	**Sodium:** 597mg	
Protein 3.61g	**Potassium** 510mg	
Vitamin A: 314IU	**Vitamin C:** 23.76mg	**Calcium:** 82mg
Iron: 1.14mg	**Thiamin:** 0.13mg	**Niacin:** 0.44mg
Vitamin B6: 0.41mg	**Magnesium:** 35mg	**Folate:** 60µg

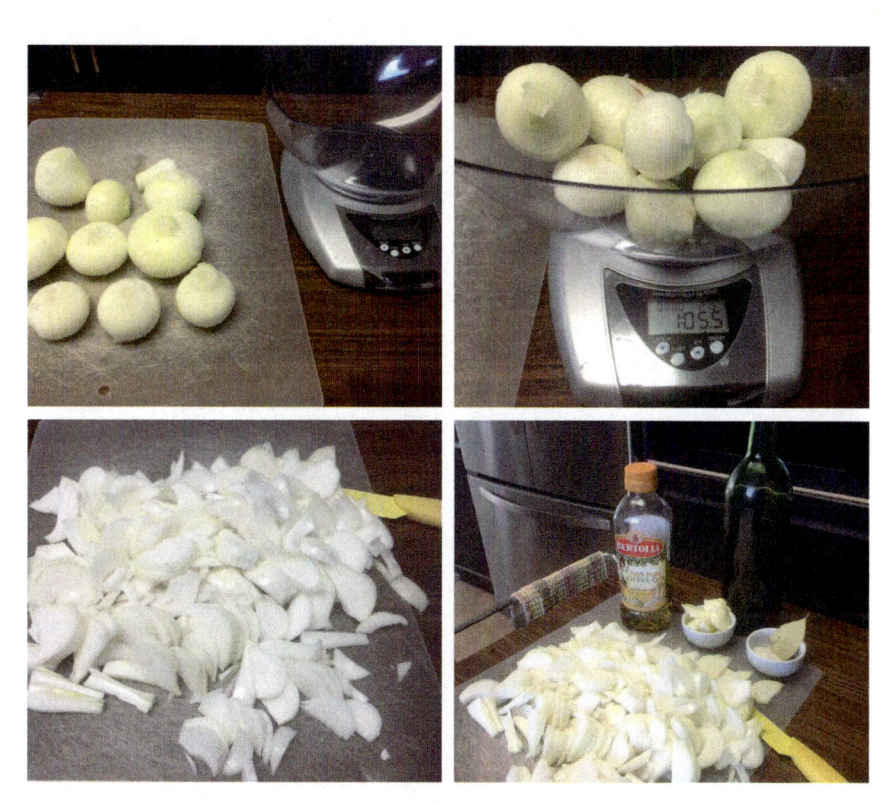

102

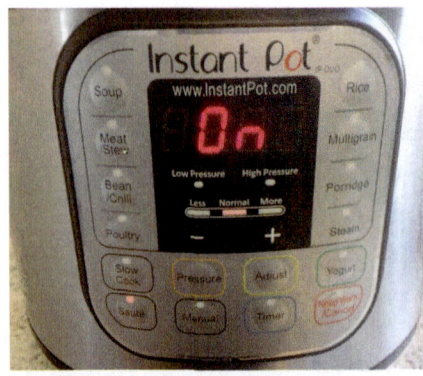

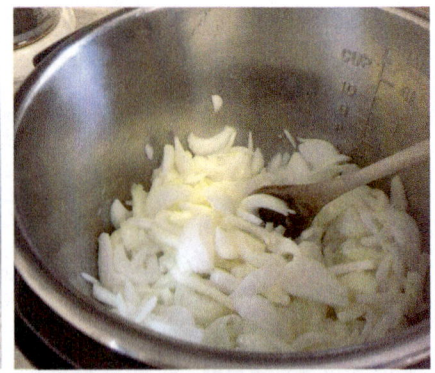

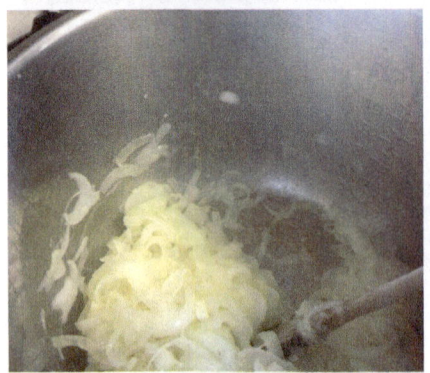

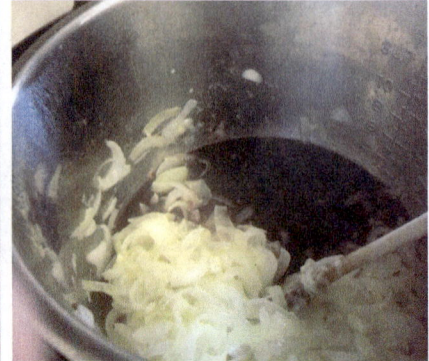

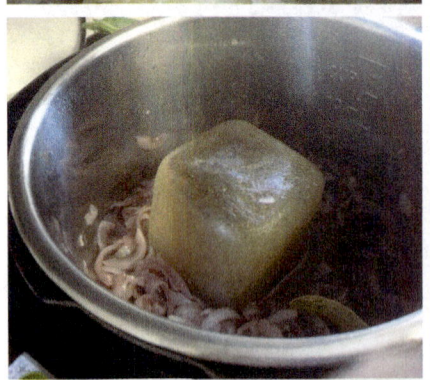

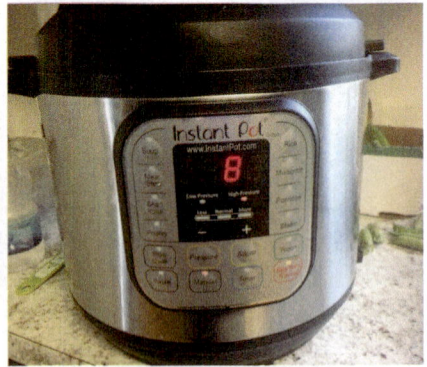

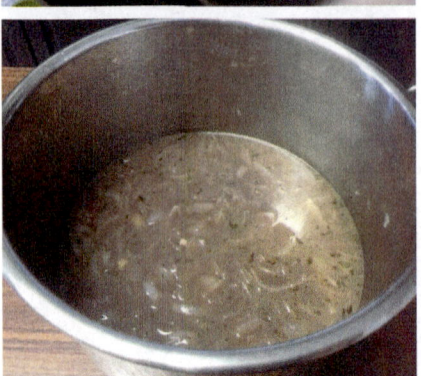

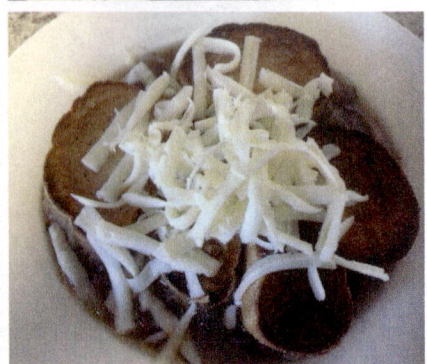

White Bean & Beet Greens Soup

Vegan	Oil-free	WFPB		Servings: 10

INGREDIENTS

- 1 medium yellow onion, chopped
- 2 medium carrots, chopped
- 2 stalks celery, chopped
- 4 cloves garlic, minced
- 1 teaspoon (5 ml) rosemary
- 1 teaspoon (5 ml) thyme
- 1 teaspoon (5 ml) poultry seasoning
- 1 teaspoon (5 ml) red pepper flakes
- 2 tablespoons (30 ml) white vinegar
- 1 tablespoon (15 ml) soy sauce
- 6 cups (1.4 L) vegetable broth, preferably homemade
- 2 cups (400g) white beans, soaked overnight
- 2 large tomatoes, chopped
- 3 cups (114g) beet greens, chopped, fresh or frozen
- 1 teaspoon (5 ml) Himalayan pink salt
- 1 teaspoon (5 ml) black pepper, freshly ground

DIRECTIONS

1. Place all of the ingredients in the inner liner of your Instant Pot and stir well.
2. Close and lock the lid, ensuring the Pressure Valve is in the Sealing position.

3. Select the Soup/Broth button and set the cooking time for 15 minutes.
4. Once cooking time is complete, allow a 10-minute NPR (Natural Pressure Release).
5. Then, release the rest of the pressure by carefully turning the Pressure Valve from Sealing to Venting.
6. When all the pressure has been released and the Float Valve has dropped, carefully remove the lid and give the soup a good stir.
7. Serve immediately or refrigerate or freeze for later use.

Useful Information on total cooking time:

Time to come to pressure: approx. 25 minutes

Cooking time: 15 minutes

NPR: 10 minutes

QR: time for pressure to release: 4 minutes

Total Instant Pot time: approx. 54 minutes

Nutritional Information per Serving:

Nutritional Information per Serving			
Servings	10		
Calories: 172		**Total fat:** 0.66g	
Calories from fat: 5 (3%)		Saturated: 0.12g	
Total Carbohydrates: 32.55g		Monounsaturated: 0.08g	
Dietary Fiber: 8.22g		Polyunsaturated: 0.45g	
Sugars: 5.09g		Trans fat: NA	
Cholesterol: --		**Sodium:** 698mg	
Protein 10.47g		**Potassium** 775mg	
Vitamin A: 3509IU	**Vitamin C:** 11.01mg	**Calcium:** 99mg	
Iron: 3.10mg	**Thiamin:** 0.36mg	**Niacin:** 1.41mg	
Vitamin B6: 0.28mg	**Magnesium:** 91mg	**Folate:** 168µg	

105

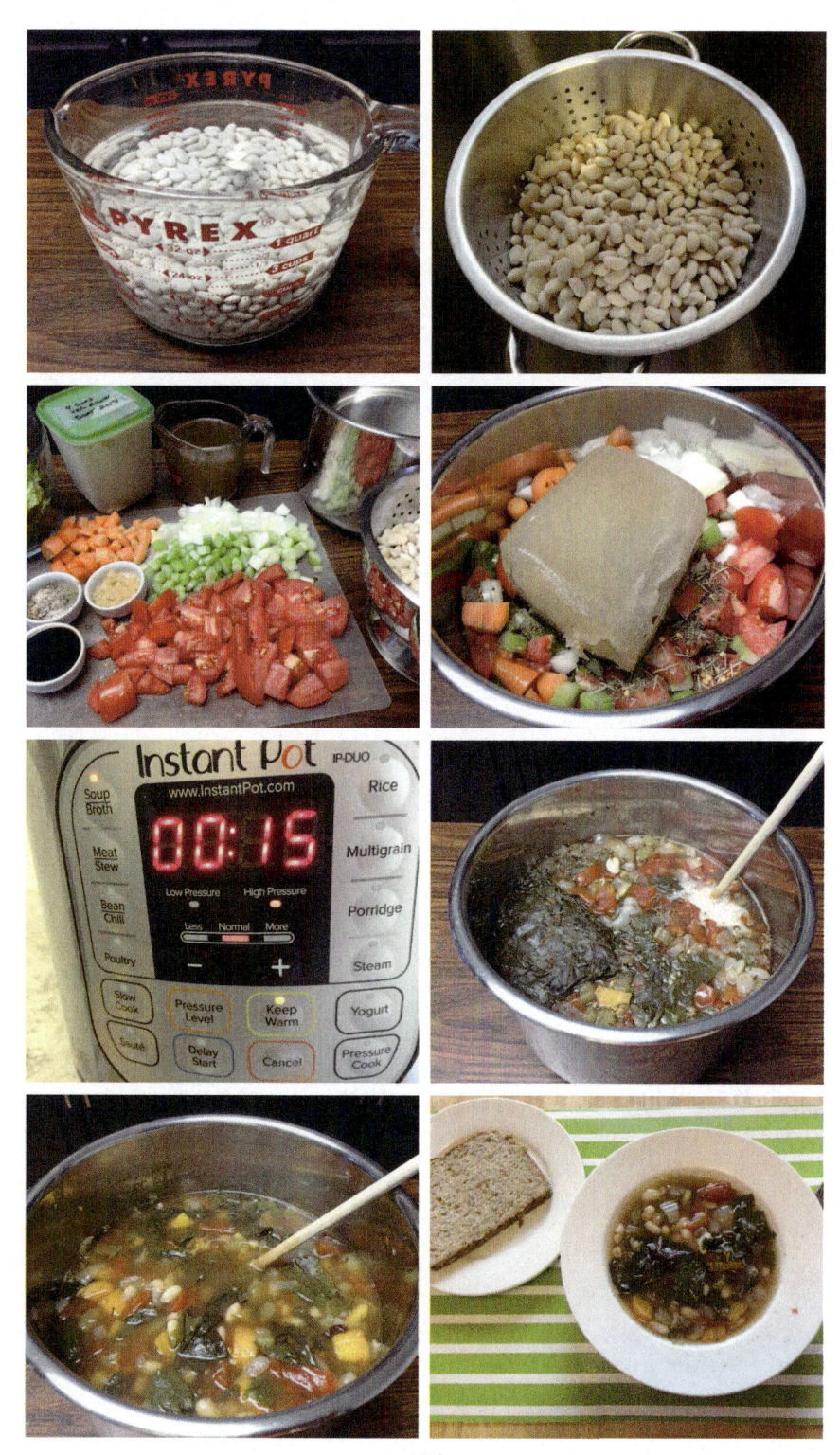

Creamy Potato Leek Soup

Vegan	Oil-free	WFPB		Servings: 8

This soup is a favorite and we make it often. If you like, you can peel the potatoes. We prefer not to as we like the extra nutrition provided by the skins. We also like our soup a little chunky so we don't blend it until it's completely smooth.

INGREDIENTS

- 3 large leeks, white parts only, washed, sliced
- 4 large potatoes, Russet, cut into chunks
- 6 cups (1.4 L) vegetable broth, preferably homemade
- 2 teaspoons (10 ml) dried thyme
- 2 bay leaves
- 1 teaspoon (5 ml) sea salt, or to taste
- 1 teaspoon (5 ml) black pepper, or to taste, freshly ground

DIRECTIONS

1. Place all of the ingredients in the inner pot of your Instant Pot, with the exception of the salt and pepper. Stir.
2. Close and lock the lid ensuring the Pressure Valve is in the Sealing position.
3. Select the Soup/Broth button and set the cooking time for 6 minutes.
4. Once cooking time is complete, allow a 10-minute Natural Pressure Release (NPR), then release the rest of the pressure by carefully turning the Pressure Valve from Sealing to Venting.

5. Once all of the pressure has been released and the Float Valve has dropped, carefully remove the lid.
6. Remove the bay leaves.
7. Purée the soup with an immersion blender until smooth. (Note: You can also use a regular blender - like a VitaMix - if you prefer - and purée the soup in batches.)
8. Add salt and pepper to taste.
9. Serve immediately or refrigerate or freeze for later use.

Nutritional Information per serving:

Nutritional Information per Serving		
Servings 8		
Calories: 177	**Total fat:** 0.27g	
Calories from fat: 2 (1%)	**Saturated:** 0.06g	
Total Carbohydrates: 40.92g	**Monounsaturated:** 0.06g	
Dietary Fiber: 3.24g	**Polyunsaturated:** 0.15g	
Sugars: 3.95g	Trans fat: NA	
Cholesterol: --	**Sodium:** 718mg	
Protein 4.59g	**Potassium** 842mg	
Vitamin A: 946IU	**Vitamin C:** 14.76mg	**Calcium:** 52mg
Iron: 2.82mg	**Thiamin:** 0.17mg	**Niacin:** 2.07mg
Vitamin B6: 0.71mg	**Magnesium:** 53mg	**Folate:** 47µg

Split Pea and Potato Soup

| Vegan | Oil-free | WFPB | | Servings: 8 |

This is another staple at our house. We love the taste of split pea soup and this is just so easy to make.

INGREDIENTS

2 cups (450g) split peas, rinsed

6 cups (1.4L) vegetable broth, preferably homemade

1 large yellow onion, chopped

4 medium red potatoes, chunked

4-6 cloves garlic, minced

3 large carrots, large dice

2 ribs celery, chopped

1 bay leaf

1 teaspoon (5 ml) smoked paprika

1 teaspoon (5 ml) basil

1 teaspoon (5 ml) thyme

2 tablespoons (30 ml) nutritional yeast

¼ teaspoon (1.25 ml) cayenne pepper

1 teaspoon (5 ml) Himalayan pink salt

DIRECTIONS

1. Prepare all the ingredients per the list of ingredients.
2. Add all the ingredients to the inner pot of the Instant Pot. Stir.
3. Close and lock the lid of the Instant Pot, ensuring that the Pressure Valve is in the Sealing Position.

4. Select the Soup/Broth button and set the cooking time for 15 minutes.
5. Once the cooking time is complete, allow a 10-minute Natural Pressure Release, then carefully turn the Pressure Valve from Sealing to Venting to release any remaining pressure. It will take approximately 5 minutes or so for the Float Valve to drop.
6. Once all the pressure has been released and the Float Valve has dropped, carefully remove the lid.
7. Then, carefully remove the inner pot to a heatproof surface.
8. Stir well and serve immediately or refrigerate or freeze for later use.

Useful Information on total cooking time:

Time to come to pressure: approx. 23-28 minutes

Cooking time: 15 minutes

NPR: 10 minutes

QR: time for pressure to release: 5 minutes

Total Instant Pot time: approx. 53-58 minutes

Nutritional Information per Serving:

Nutritional Information per Serving	
Servings 8	
Calories: 308	**Total fat:** 0.66g
Calories from fat: 5 (1%)	Saturated: 0.14g
Total Carbohydrates: 60.81g	Monounsaturated: 0.14g
Dietary Fiber: 16.20g	Polyunsaturated: 0.38g
Sugars: 9.20g	Trans fat: NA
Cholesterol: --	**Sodium:** 888mg
Protein 16.23g	**Potassium** 1186mg
Vitamin A: 5220IU	**Vitamin C:** 19.34mg	**Calcium:** 75mg
Iron: 3.84mg	**Thiamin:** 1.52mg	**Niacin:** 9.00mg
Vitamin B6: 0.50mg	**Magnesium:** 67mg	**Folate:** 343µg

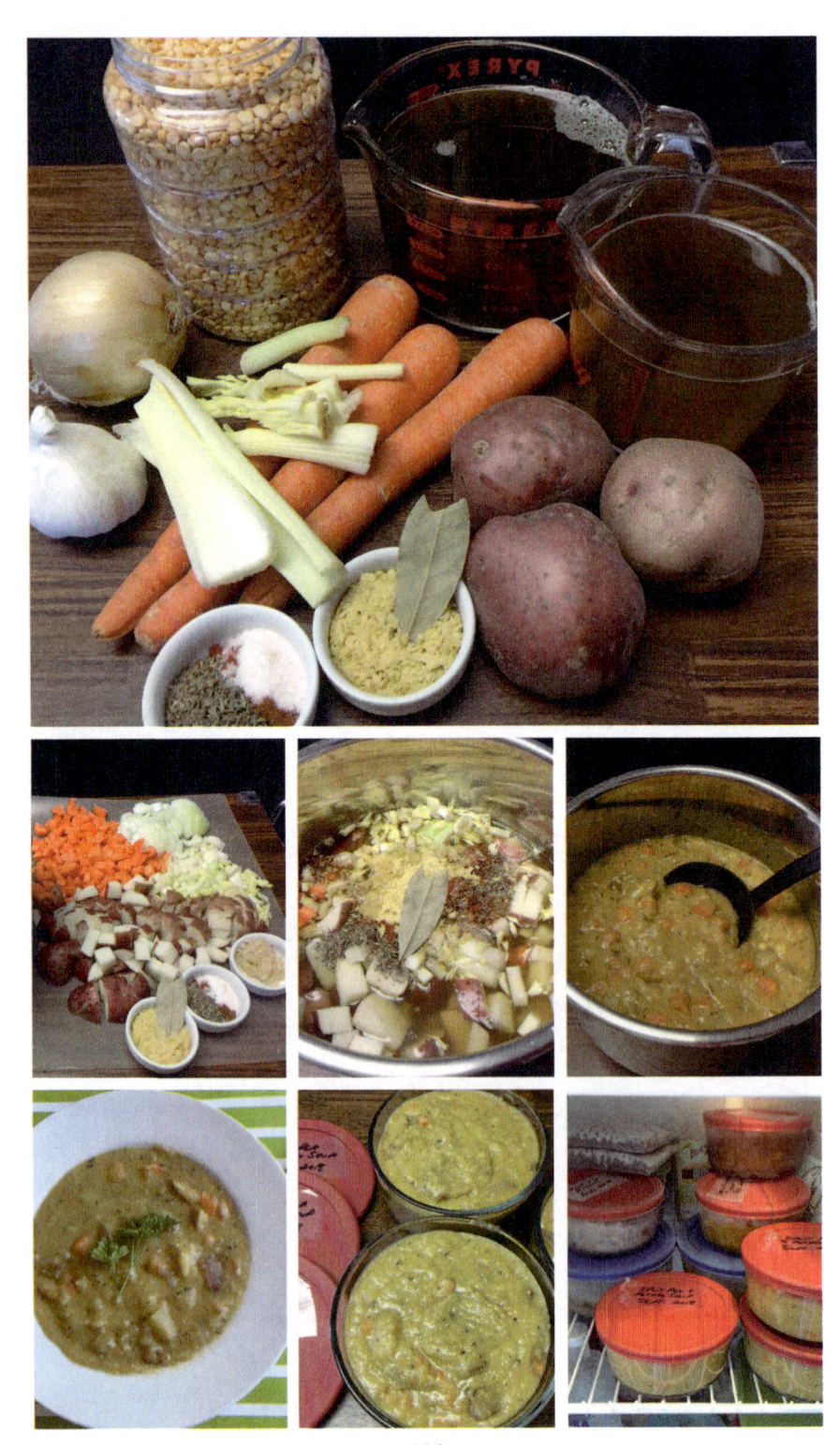

Mung Bean Soup

Vegan	Oil-free	WFPB		Servings: 8

We usually have a lot of mung beans in the house because we also use them for making bean sprouts for our stir fries. However, they are lovely in a soup and can be cooked from dry as we did in this recipe.

INGREDIENTS

2 cups (400g) dried mung beans

2 medium onions, chopped

2 large carrots, chopped

2 stalks celery, sliced

4 cloves garlic, minced

1 tablespoon (15 ml) water

¼ cup (60 ml) tomato paste

6 cups (1.4 L) vegetable broth

4 cups (950 ml) tomato juice

1 tablespoon (15 ml) Herbes de Provence, or Italian seasoning

2 teaspoons (10 ml) sea salt, or to taste

1 teaspoon (5 ml) black pepper, freshly ground, to taste

½ teaspoon (2.5 ml) red pepper flakes, optional

DIRECTIONS

1. Prepare all the ingredients per the list of ingredients.
2. Add all the ingredients to the inner pot of the Instant Pot. Stir.
3. Close and lock the lid of the Instant Pot, ensuring that the Pressure Valve is in the Sealing Position.

4. Select the Soup/Broth button and set the cooking time for 20 minutes.
5. Once the cooking time is complete, allow a full Natural Pressure Release. This means just letting your Instant Pot sit (you can let it stay on Keep Warm or you can push the Cancel button) until the Float Valve drops on its own.
6. Once the Float Valve has dropped, carefully remove the lid.
7. Then, carefully remove the inner pot to a heatproof surface.
8. Stir well and serve immediately or refrigerate or freeze for later use.

Nutritional Information per Serving:

Nutritional Information per Serving			
Servings	8		
Calories: 229		**Total fat:** 0.51g	
Calories from fat: 4 (2%)		Saturated: 0.17g	
Total Carbohydrates: 44.52g		Monounsaturated: 0.07g	
Dietary Fiber: 10.15g		Polyunsaturated: 0.28g	
Sugars: 8.99g		Trans fat: NA	
Cholesterol: --		**Sodium:** 1045mg	
Protein 13.97g		**Potassium** 1413mg	
Vitamin A: 4186IU		**Vitamin C:** 91.14mg	**Calcium:** 169mg
Iron: 6.45mg		**Thiamin:** 0.37mg	**Niacin:** 1.62mg
Vitamin B6: 0.36mg		**Magnesium:** 121mg	**Folate:** 236µg

Lima Bean Soup

Vegan	Oil-free	WFPB		Servings: 8

Not everyone likes lima beans but we sure do. If they're not on your list of favorites, you can try substituting a different bean but the flavor won't be the same and, depending on the bean, you may need to adjust the cooking time.

INGREDIENTS

16 ounces (454g) dried baby Lima beans, (approx. 2 cups)

1 medium yellow onion, chopped

2 medium carrots, chopped

1 rib celery, chopped

3 cloves garlic, minced

4 cups (950 ml) vegetable broth

1 teaspoon (5 ml) poultry seasoning

1 medium bay leaf

1 teaspoon (5 ml) sea salt

1 cup (100g) baby spinach, packed

DIRECTIONS

1. Prepare all the ingredients per the list of ingredients.
2. Add all the ingredients to the inner pot of the Instant Pot with the exception of the baby spinach.
3. Close and lock the lid of the Instant Pot, ensuring that the Pressure Valve is in the Sealing Position.
4. Select the Bean/Chili button and set the cooking time for 30 minutes.

5. Once the cooking time is complete, allow a 30-minute Natural Pressure Release, then carefully turn the Pressure Valve from Sealing to Venting to release any remaining pressure. It will take approximately 5 minutes or so for the Float Valve to drop.
6. Once all the pressure has been released and the Float Valve has dropped, carefully remove the lid and remove the inner pot to a heatproof surface.
7. Add the baby spinach and stir well until the spinach has wilted. Serve immediately or refrigerate or freeze for later use.

Nutritional Information per Serving:

Nutritional Information per Serving		
Servings 8		
Calories: 211	**Total fat:** 0.47g	
Calories from fat: 4 (2%)	**Saturated:** 0.14g	
Total Carbohydrates: 40.79g	**Monounsaturated:** 0.05g	
Dietary Fiber: 12.61g	**Polyunsaturated:** 0.28g	
Sugars: 7.16g	**Trans fat:** NA	
Cholesterol: --	**Sodium:** 593mg	
Protein 12.24g	**Potassium** 911mg	
Vitamin A: 3195IU	**Vitamin C:** 3.63mg	**Calcium:** 65mg
Iron: 3.82mg	**Thiamin:** 0.34mg	**Niacin:** 1.20mg
Vitamin B6: 0.25mg	**Magnesium:** 114mg	**Folate:** 242µg

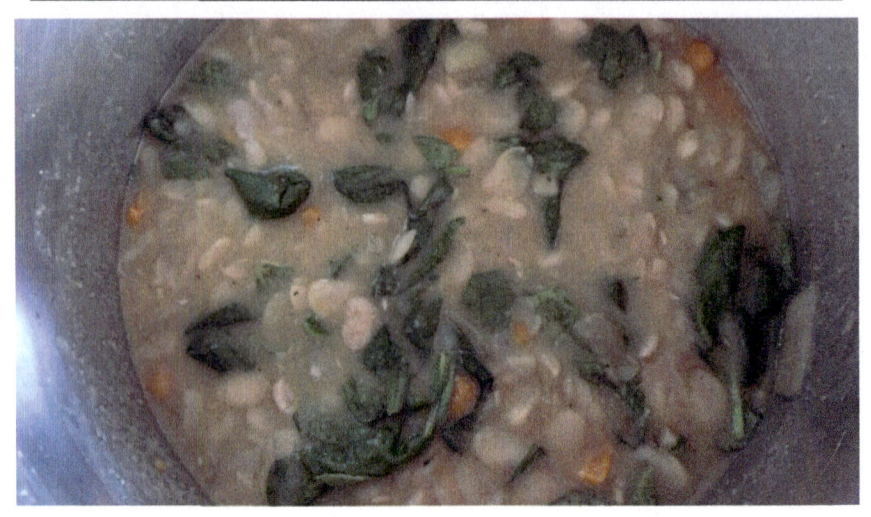

Minestrone Soup

| Vegan | Oil-free | WFPB | | Servings: 12 |

Positively packed with protein, this soup is hearty enough to serve as a meal with some crusty bread on the side. This Instant Pot version is easy to make and you can freeze any leftovers for later use.

INGREDIENTS

7 cups (1.65 L) vegetable broth, preferably homemade

1½ cups (150g) pasta of your choice

1 medium yellow onion, chopped

2 large carrots, chopped

1 stalk celery, sliced

1 medium zucchini, chopped

4 cloves garlic, minced

1½ cups (255g) kidney beans, or beans of your choice, canned or home cooked

1½ teaspoons (7.5 ml) oregano

1½ teaspoons (7.5 ml) rosemary

1 teaspoon (5 ml) tarragon

1 teaspoon (5 ml) thyme

1 teaspoon (5 ml) sea salt

1 teaspoon (5 ml) pepper, freshly ground

3½ cups (795g) diced tomatoes, canned

2 cups (200g) baby spinach, or beet greens

DIRECTIONS

1. Add all of the ingredients to the inner liner of your Instant Pot in the order given, with the exception of the spinach, making sure the pasta is completely covered by the liquid.
2. DO NOT STIR. This is because you want the other ingredients to hold the pasta under the liquid so it cooks properly.
3. Close and lock the lid, ensuring that the Pressure Valve is in the Sealing position.
4. Select the Soup/Broth mode and set the cooking time for 4 minutes.
5. Once the cooking time is complete, allow a 5-minute Natural Pressure Release (this allows the contents to "settle down" a bit before you release the pressure).
6. Then, release the remaining pressure by carefully turning the Pressure Valve from Sealing to Venting.
7. When all the pressure has been released, carefully remove the lid and then transfer the inner pot to a heatproof surface.
8. Add the spinach and give the soup a good stir.
9. Serve immediately, or refrigerate or freeze for later use.

Useful Information on total cooking time:

Time to come to pressure: approx. 30 minutes

Cooking time: 4 minutes

NPR: 5 minutes

QR: time for pressure to release: approx. 5 minutes

Total Instant Pot time: approx. 44 minutes

Nutritional Information per Serving:

Nutritional Information per Serving	
Servings 12	
Calories: 403	**Total fat:** 2.18g
Calories from fat: 19 (4%)	Saturated: 0.51g
Total Carbohydrates: 81.82g	Monounsaturated: 0.68g
Dietary Fiber: 14.08g	Polyunsaturated: 0.99g
Sugars: 19.88g	Trans fat: NA
Cholesterol: --	**Sodium:** 1464mg
Protein 18.32g	**Potassium** 1461mg
Vitamin A: 3532IU	**Vitamin C:** 36.80mg	**Calcium:** 197mg
Iron: 7.95mg	**Thiamin:** 0.81mg	**Niacin:** 8.06mg
Vitamin B6: 0.72mg	**Magnesium:** 133mg	**Folate:** 220µg

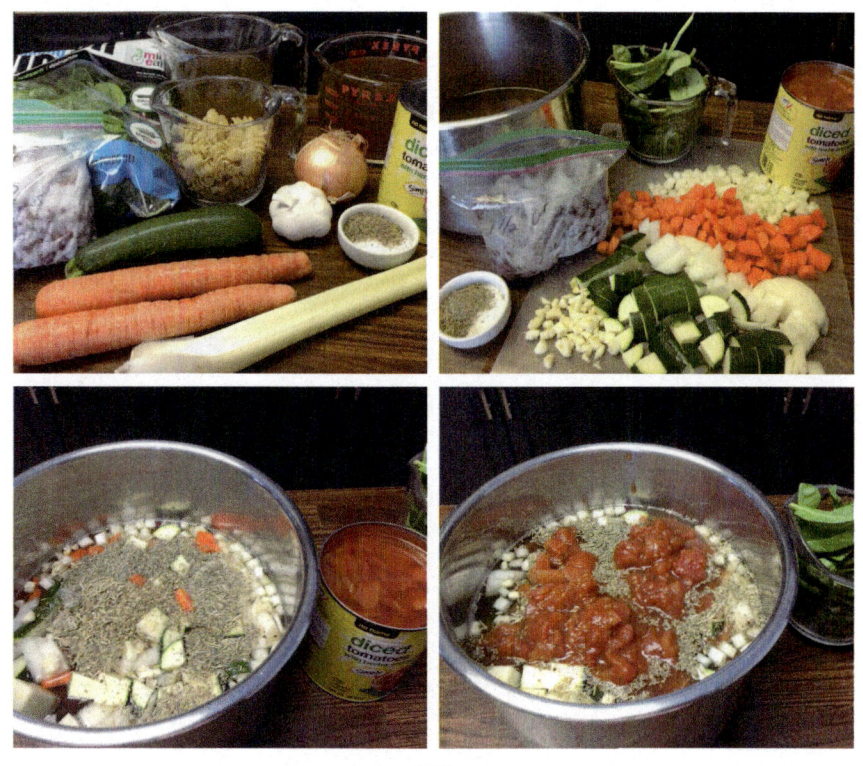

118

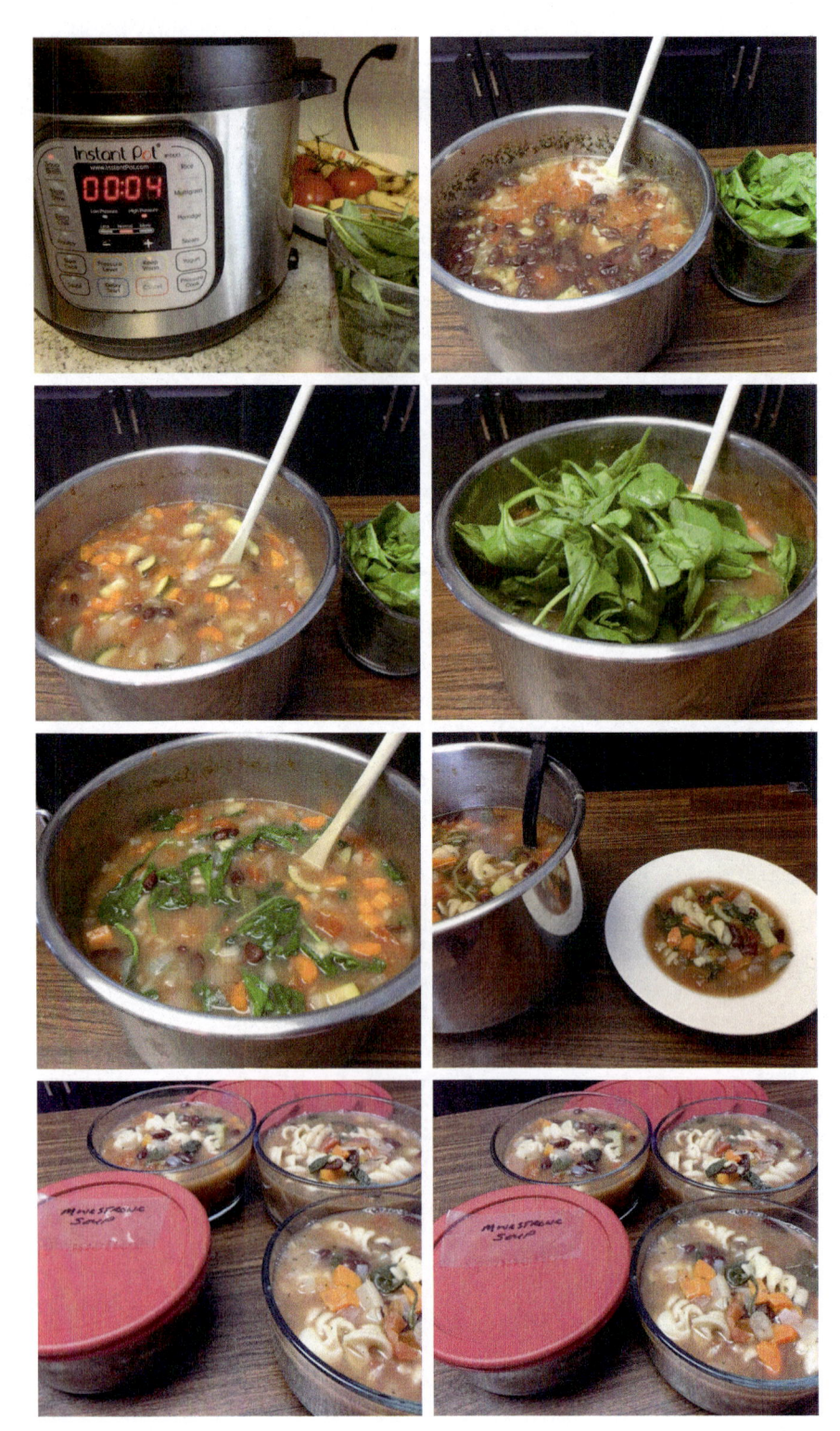

Instant Pot Mulligatawny Soup

| Vegan | Oil-free | WFPB | | Servings: 6 |

Mulligatawny sounds like it should be Irish but then you discover it contains curry so now you think it's Indian. Well that's sort of right but mulligatawny is actually an English soup based on a Tamil recipe. You can look up more info on Wikipedia.

This soup is frequently made with chicken but this is the vegan version.

INGREDIENTS

2 carrots, peeled and roughly chopped

2 onions, roughly chopped

1 stalk celery, roughly chopped

3 slices ginger (about quarter size) peeled

5 cloves garlic, roughly chopped

2 tablespoons (30 ml) curry powder

1 teaspoon (5 ml) ground coriander

6 cups (1.4 L) vegetable broth, homemade if possible

1 medium baking potato, scrubbed but unpeeled, roughly chopped

¾ cup (180 ml) coconut milk

2 tablespoons (30 ml) lime juice, fresh if possible

3 tablespoons (45 ml) fresh cilantro, chopped (optional)

DIRECTIONS

1. Add all of the ingredients to the inner liner of your Instant Pot with the exception of the coconut milk, lime juice and cilantro.

2. Close and lock the lid ensuring that the Pressure Valve is in the Sealing position.
3. Select the Soup/Broth button and set the cooking time for 18 minutes.
4. Once cooking time is complete, allow a Natural Pressure Release for 10 minutes and then manually release the rest of the pressure by carefully turning the Pressure Valve from Sealing to Venting.
5. When all of the pressure has been released and the Float Valve has dropped, carefully remove the lid.
6. Carefully remove the inner liner to a heatproof surface.
7. Using an immersion blender, blend the soup until smooth, then add the coconut milk and lime juice and stir well.
8. Serve immediately, using the chopped cilantro as a garnish, if desired.

Nutritional Information per Serving:

Nutritional Information per Serving		
Servings 6		
Calories: 133	**Total fat:** 6.11g	
Calories from fat: 54 (41%)	Saturated: 5.42g	
Total Carbohydrates: 18.85g	Monounsaturated: 0.49g	
Dietary Fiber: 3.60g	Polyunsaturated: 0.19g	
Sugars: 5.30g	Trans fat: NA	
Cholesterol: --	**Sodium:** 583mg	
Protein 2.54g	**Potassium** 420mg	
Vitamin A: 4595IU	**Vitamin C:** 14.30mg	**Calcium:** 48mg
Iron: 1.89mg	**Thiamin:** 0.08mg	**Niacin:** 0.97mg
Vitamin B6: 0.23mg	**Magnesium:** 35mg	**Folate:** 26μg

Useful Information on total cooking time:
(We used semi-frozen vegetable broth.)

Time to come to pressure: approx. 27 minutes

Cooking time: 18 minutes

NPR: 10 minutes

QR: time for pressure to release: approx. 2 minutes

Total Instant Pot time: approx. 57 minutes

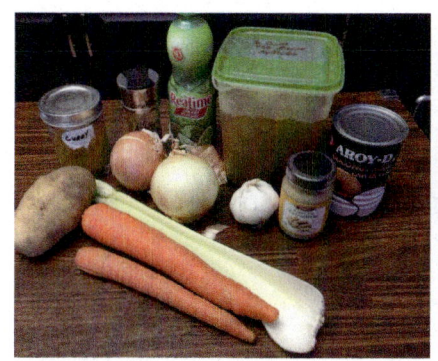

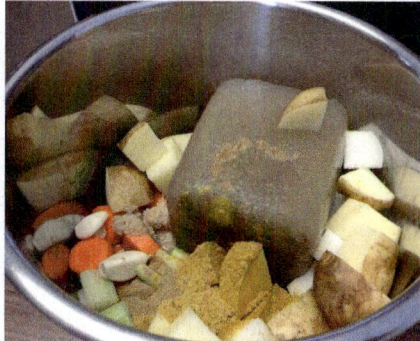

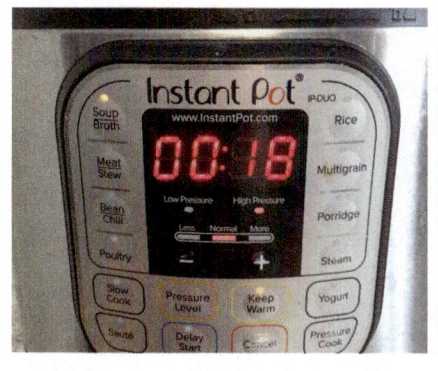

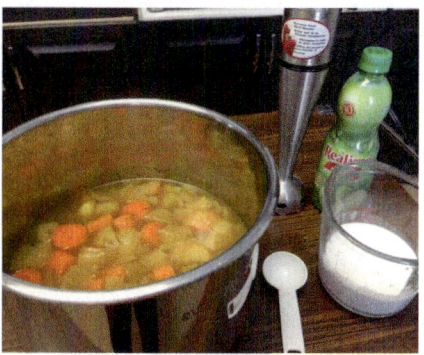

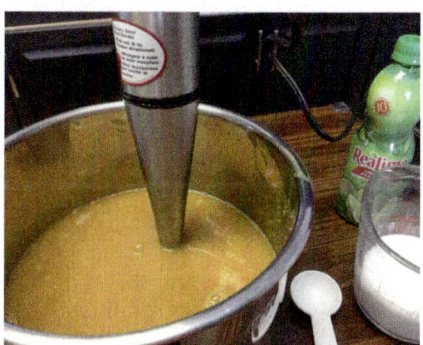

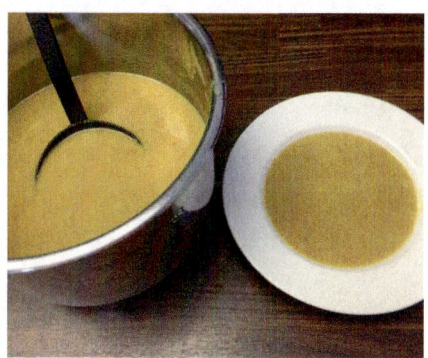

Simple Cabbage Soup

| Vegan | Oil-free | WFPB | | Servings: 8 |

Super low-calorie. Easy to make.

INGREDIENTS

4 cups (400g) green cabbage, chopped

3 cups (300g) baby spinach

2 large carrots, chopped

2 large celery stalks, sliced

2 small yellow onions, chopped

2 medium tomatoes, chopped

½ cup (120 ml) crushed tomatoes

3 cloves garlic, minced

1½ teaspoons (7.5 ml) sea salt, or to taste

1½ teaspoons (7.5 ml) basil

1½ teaspoons (7.5 ml) oregano

½ teaspoon (2.5 ml) red pepper flakes

4 cups (950 ml) vegetable broth

DIRECTIONS

1. Prepare all the ingredients per the list of ingredients.
2. Add all the ingredients to the inner pot of the Instant Pot.
3. Close and lock the lid of the Instant Pot, ensuring that the Pressure Valve is in the Sealing Position.
4. Select the Soup/Broth button and set the cooking time for 4 minutes.

5. Once the cooking time is complete, allow a 10-minute Natural Pressure Release, then carefully turn the Pressure Valve from Sealing to Venting to release any remaining pressure. It will take approximately 5 minutes or so for the Float Valve to drop.
6. Once all the pressure has been released and the Float Valve has dropped, carefully remove the lid.
7. Then, carefully remove the inner pot to a heatproof surface.
8. Stir well and serve immediately or refrigerate or freeze for later use.

Nutritional Information per Serving:

Nutritional Information per Serving

Servings: 8

Calories: 49	**Total fat:** 0.21g
Calories from fat: 1 (3%)	Saturated: 0.06g
Total Carbohydrates: 11.30g	Monounsaturated: 0.03g
Dietary Fiber: 3.27g	Polyunsaturated: 0.11g
Sugars: 5.79g	Trans fat: NA

Cholesterol: --	**Sodium:** 783mg
Protein 2.00g	**Potassium** 391mg

Vitamin A: 4773IU	**Vitamin C:** 28.37mg	**Calcium:** 61mg
Iron: 1.08mg	**Thiamin:** 0.08mg	**Niacin:** 0.83mg
Vitamin B6: 0.20mg	**Magnesium:** 27mg	**Folate:** 60µg

Garlic Soup

| Vegetarian | Oil-free | | | Servings: 8 |

Feel free to add more garlic to this recipe if you like. We often do.

INGREDIENTS

- 4 cups (950 ml) vegetable broth, preferably homemade
- 1 large parsnip, chopped (about one cup)
- 1 medium yellow onion, chopped
- 1 teaspoon (5 ml) thyme
- 1 teaspoon (5 ml) basil
- 1 teaspoon (5 ml) oregano
- 6 peppercorns
- 3 tablespoons (45 ml) garlic, chopped
- 2 teaspoons (10 ml) sea salt, to taste
- 2 ounces (55g) cheddar cheese, extra old, shredded (omit for vegan or substitute a vegan cheese)
- 2 teaspoons (10 ml) lemon juice, freshly squeezed

DIRECTIONS

1. Combine all the ingredients in your Instant Pot with the exception of the salt, lemon juice and cheese. (they will be added later)
2. Close and lock the lid ensuring the Pressure Valve is in the Sealing position.
3. Select the Soup/Broth button and set the cooking time for 5 minutes.
4. Once the cooking time is complete do a QR (Quick Release) by carefully turning the Pressure Valve from Sealing to Venting.

5. When all of the pressure has been released and the Float Valve has dropped, carefully remove the lid.
6. Add the cheese and stir well.
7. Purée until smooth using an immersion blender or by transferring the soup to a Vitamix™.
8. Add salt and lemon juice to taste.
9. Serve immediately or refrigerate or freeze for later use.

Nutritional Information per Serving:

Nutritional Information per Serving		
Servings 8		
Calories: 63	**Total fat:** 2.20g	
Calories from fat: 19 (31%)	Saturated: 1.43g	
Total Carbohydrates: 8.64g	Monounsaturated: 0.63g	
Dietary Fiber: 1.81g	Polyunsaturated: 0.14g	
Sugars: 2.49g	Trans fat: NA	
Cholesterol: 7mg	**Sodium:** 904mg	
Protein 2.52g	**Potassium** 134mg	
Vitamin A: 344IU	**Vitamin C:** 5.41mg	**Calcium:** 78mg
Iron: 0.65mg	**Thiamin:** 0.03mg	**Niacin:** 0.20mg
Vitamin B6: 0.08mg	**Magnesium:** 13mg	**Folate:** 16µg

SAUCE RECIPES

Red Lentil Mushroom Ragu

Vegan	Oil-free	WFPB		Servings: 6

Although this recipe is for 6 servings, we find it often goes much further than that. So, at only 311 calories per serving, if you stretch it further, then that, naturally, reduces the calories/serving.

INGREDIENTS

4 cups (950 ml) vegetable broth

1 large yellow onion, diced

2 stalks celery, diced

3 medium carrots, diced

12 ounces (340g) Cremini mushrooms, quartered

4 cloves garlic, diced

1½ cups (300g) red lentils, rinsed

1½ teaspoons (7.5 ml) sea salt

2 teaspoons (10 ml) thyme

2 teaspoons (10 ml) oregano

1 teaspoon (5 ml) basil

¼ teaspoon (1.25 ml) red pepper flakes

28 ounces (795g) crushed tomatoes, canned

28 ounces (795g) diced tomatoes, canned

3 tablespoons (45 ml) tomato paste

DIRECTIONS

1. Prepare all the ingredients per the list of ingredients.

2. Add all the ingredients, in the order given, to the inner liner of your Instant Pot.
3. DO NOT STIR and make sure the broth is on the BOTTOM. If the tomatoes are in contact with the bottom, you could get a "BURN NOTICE" on your Instant Pot. We know this from experience.
4. Close and lock the lid ensuring the Pressure Valve is in the Sealing Position.
5. Select the Pressure Cook/Manual button and set the cooking time for 2 minutes.
6. Once the cooking time is complete, allow a 5-minute Natural Pressure Release, then carefully turn the Pressure Valve from Sealing to Venting to release any remaining pressure.
7. Once all the pressure has been released and the Float Valve has dropped, carefully remove the lid.
8. Then, carefully remove the inner pot to a heatproof surface.
9. Stir well and serve immediately or refrigerate or freeze for later use.

Nutritional Information per Serving:

Nutritional Information per Serving			
Servings	6		
Calories: 311		**Total fat:** 1.12g	
Calories from fat: 10 (3%)		Saturated: 0.25g	
Total Carbohydrates: 62.96g		Monounsaturated: 0.22g	
Dietary Fiber: 12.94g		Polyunsaturated: 0.65g	
Sugars: 18.75g		Trans fat: NA	
Cholesterol: --		**Sodium:** 3040mg	
Protein 18.87g		**Potassium** 1645mg	
Vitamin A: 6297IU	**Vitamin C:** 33.51mg	**Calcium:** 166mg
Iron: 8.07mg	**Thiamin:** 0.70mg	**Niacin:** 7.34mg
Vitamin B6: 0.86mg	**Magnesium:** 94mg	**Folate:** 299µg

129

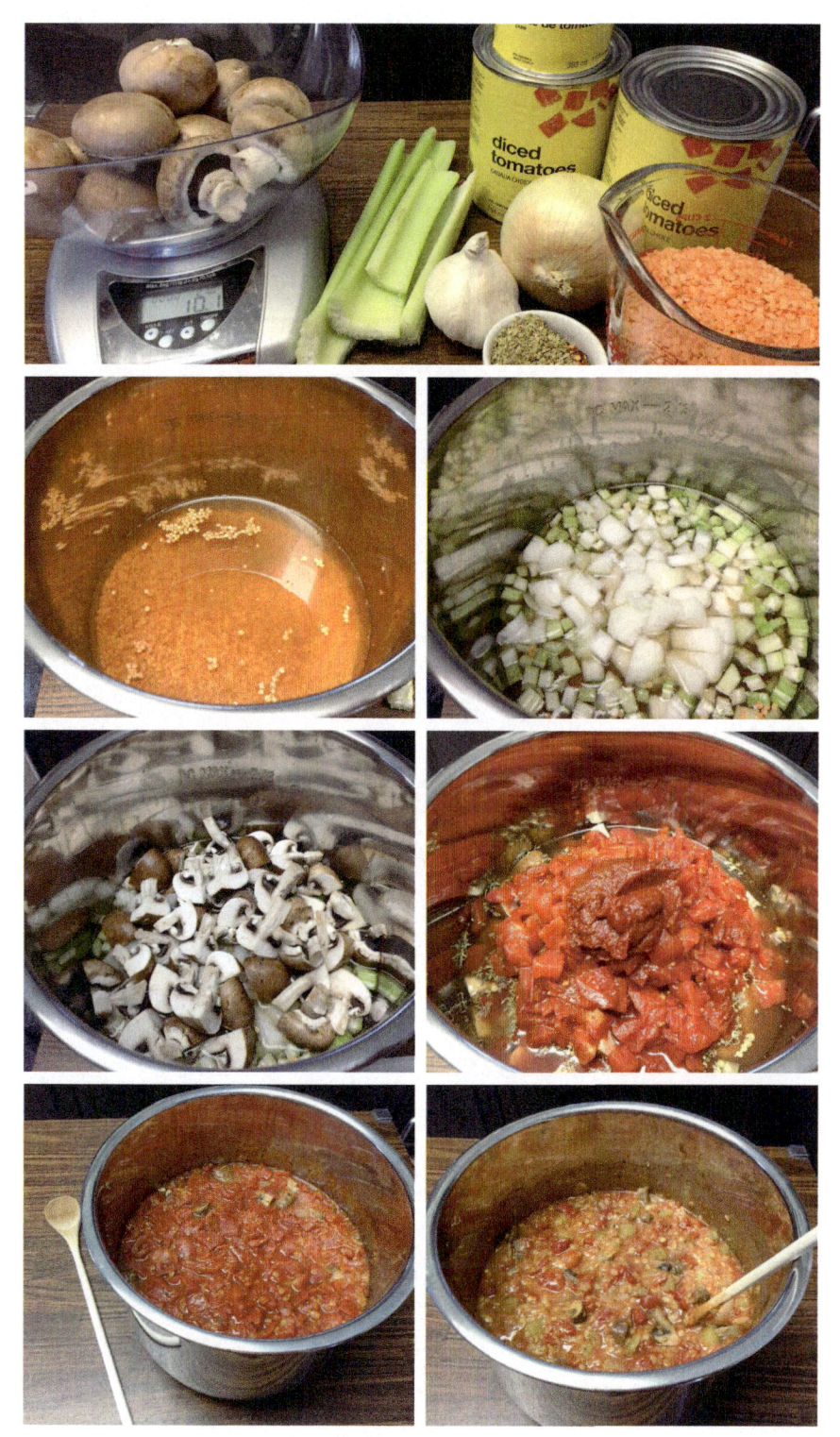

Fresh Tomato Marinara Sauce

| Vegan | Oil-free | | Servings: 20* |

*½ cup servings

One of our favorite sauces to use on pasta. We often make this in late summer or early fall when we can get Roma tomatoes by the case.

INGREDIENTS

4½ pounds (2 Kg) Roma (plum) tomatoes, diced

1 medium yellow onion, chopped

8 cloves garlic, minced

1 bay leaf

1 cup (240 ml) red wine

2 tablespoons (25g) sugar, can substitute honey if you wish but it won't be vegan

2 tablespoons (30 ml) dried basil

1 tablespoon (15 ml) dried oregano

1 tablespoon (15 ml) dried thyme

1 tablespoon (15 ml) sea salt

1 teaspoon (5 ml) black pepper, freshly ground

2 tablespoons (30 ml) balsamic vinegar

DIRECTIONS

1. Combine all of the ingredients, with the exception of the balsamic vinegar, in the inner pot of your Instant Pot and stir well.
2. Close and lock the lid ensuring the Pressure Valve is in the Sealing position.

3. Select Pressure Cook/Manual mode and set the cooking time for 5 minutes.
4. When cooking time is complete do a 10-minute Natural Pressure Release followed by a Quick Release by carefully turning the Pressure Valve from Sealing to Venting.
5. Once all the pressure has been released and the Float Valve has dropped, carefully remove the lid.
6. Add the vinegar and stir well.
7. Carefully remove the inner pot to a heatproof surface and blend with an immersion blender until smooth. If you don't have an immersion blender, you can use a regular blender and blend the sauce in batches until smooth.
8. Transfer the sauce to sterilized canning jars and allow to cool.
9. Refrigerate or freeze for later use.

Note: If you decide to freeze your sauce, you may want to consider using plastic containers or bags. We have experienced glass containers cracking in the freezer.

Nutritional Information per Serving

Nutritional Information per Serving			
Servings	20		
Calories: 106		**Total fat:** 0.65g	
Calories from fat: 5 (5%)		Saturated: 0.12g	
Total Carbohydrates: 21.41g		Monounsaturated: 0.15g	
Dietary Fiber: 6.07g		Polyunsaturated: 0.38g	
Sugars: 14.05g		Trans fat: NA	
Cholesterol: --		**Sodium:** 373mg	
Protein 4.40g		**Potassium** 1149mg	
Vitamin A: 3888IU	**Vitamin C:** 64.57mg	**Calcium:** 69mg	
Iron: 2.05mg	**Thiamin:** 0.15mg	**Niacin:** 2.83mg	
Vitamin B6: 0.41mg	**Magnesium:** 57mg	**Folate:** 73μg	

Note: You can also can this sauce, if you prefer, using the water bath or steam method. How to can them is beyond the scope of this book. For more information on safe home canning, you may want to visit the National Center for Home Food Preservation at:

https://nchfp.uga.edu/publications/publications_usda.html

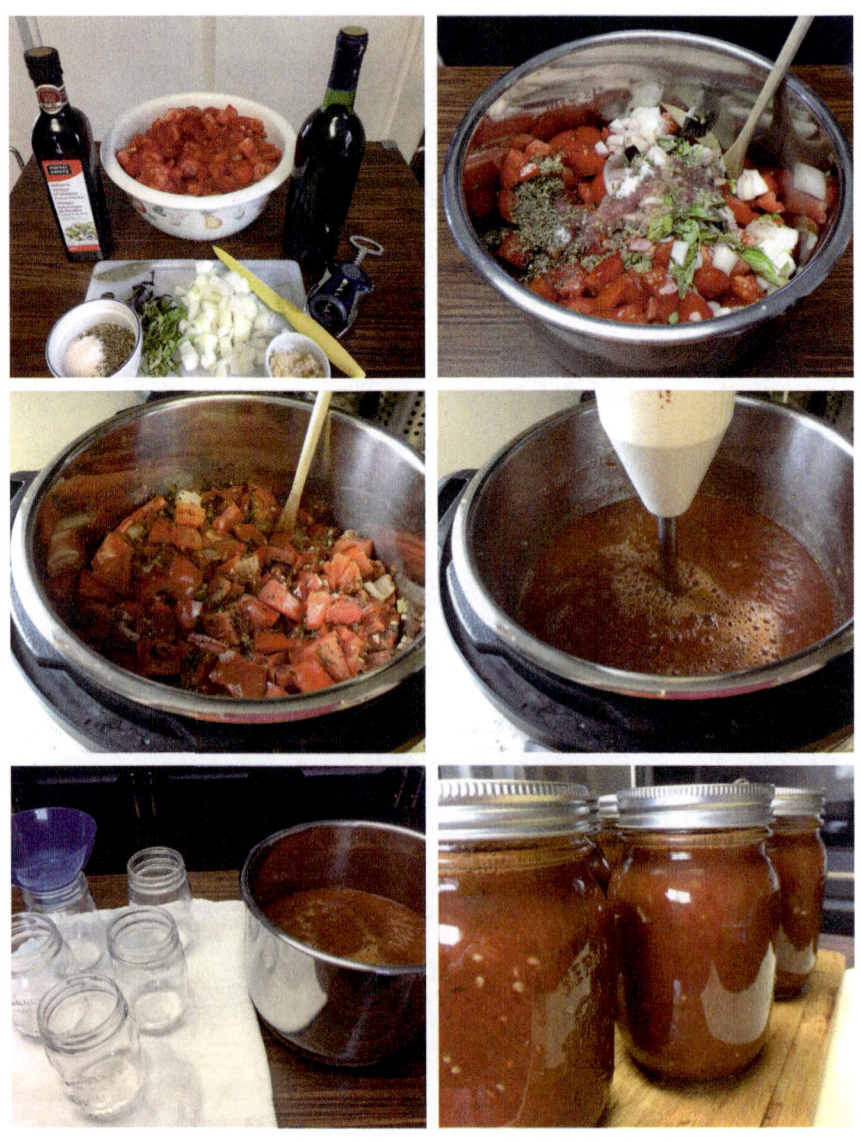

Fresh Tomato Basil Sauce

Vegan	Oil-free	WFPB		Servings: 20*

*½ cup servings

This sauce works well for any pasta dish or as an ingredient in other recipes, too.

INGREDIENTS

4½ pounds (2 Kg) Roma (plum) tomatoes, diced

1 medium yellow onion, diced

8 cloves garlic, minced

1 tablespoon (15 ml) sea salt

½ teaspoon (2.5 ml) black pepper, freshly ground

1½ teaspoons (7.5 ml) marjoram, dried

1½ teaspoons (7.5 ml) oregano, dried

¼ teaspoon (1.25 ml) crushed red pepper

1 medium bay leaf

¼ cup (6g) fresh basil, chopped

¼ cup (15g) fresh parsley, chopped

DIRECTIONS

1. Combine all of the ingredients in the inner pot of your Instant Pot and stir well.
2. Close and lock the lid ensuring the Pressure Valve is in the Sealing position.
3. Select Pressure Cook/Manual mode and set the cooking time for 8 minutes.

4. When cooking time is complete do a Quick Release by carefully turning the Pressure Valve from Sealing to Venting.
5. Once all the pressure has been released and the Float Valve has dropped, carefully remove the lid.
6. Stir well.
7. Carefully remove the inner pot to a heatproof surface and blend with an immersion blender until smooth. If you don't have an immersion blender, you can use a regular blender and blend the sauce in batches until smooth.
8. Transfer the sauce to sterilized canning jars and allow to cool.
9. Refrigerate or freeze for later use.

> *Note: If you decide to freeze your sauce, you may want to consider using plastic containers or bags. We have experienced glass containers cracking in the freezer.*

> *Note: You can also can this sauce, if you prefer, using the water bath or steam method. How to can them is beyond the scope of this book. For more information on safe home canning, you may want to visit the National Center for Home Food Preservation at:*

> https://nchfp.uga.edu/publications/publications_usda.html

Nutritional Information per Serving:

Nutritional Information per Serving		
Servings	26	
Calories: 35	**Total fat:** 0.23g	
Calories from fat: 2 (5%)	Saturated: 0.06g	
Total Carbohydrates: 8.07g	Monounsaturated: 0.05g	
Dietary Fiber: 2.51g	Polyunsaturated: 0.12g	
Sugars: 3.84g	Trans fat: NA	
Cholesterol: --	**Sodium:** 1483mg	
Protein 1.49g	**Potassium** 319mg	
Vitamin A: 1044IU	**Vitamin C:** 16.97mg	**Calcium:** 50mg
Iron: 1.09mg	**Thiamin:** 0.05mg	**Niacin:** 0.75mg
Vitamin B6: 0.15mg	**Magnesium:** 20mg	**Folate:** 26µg

135

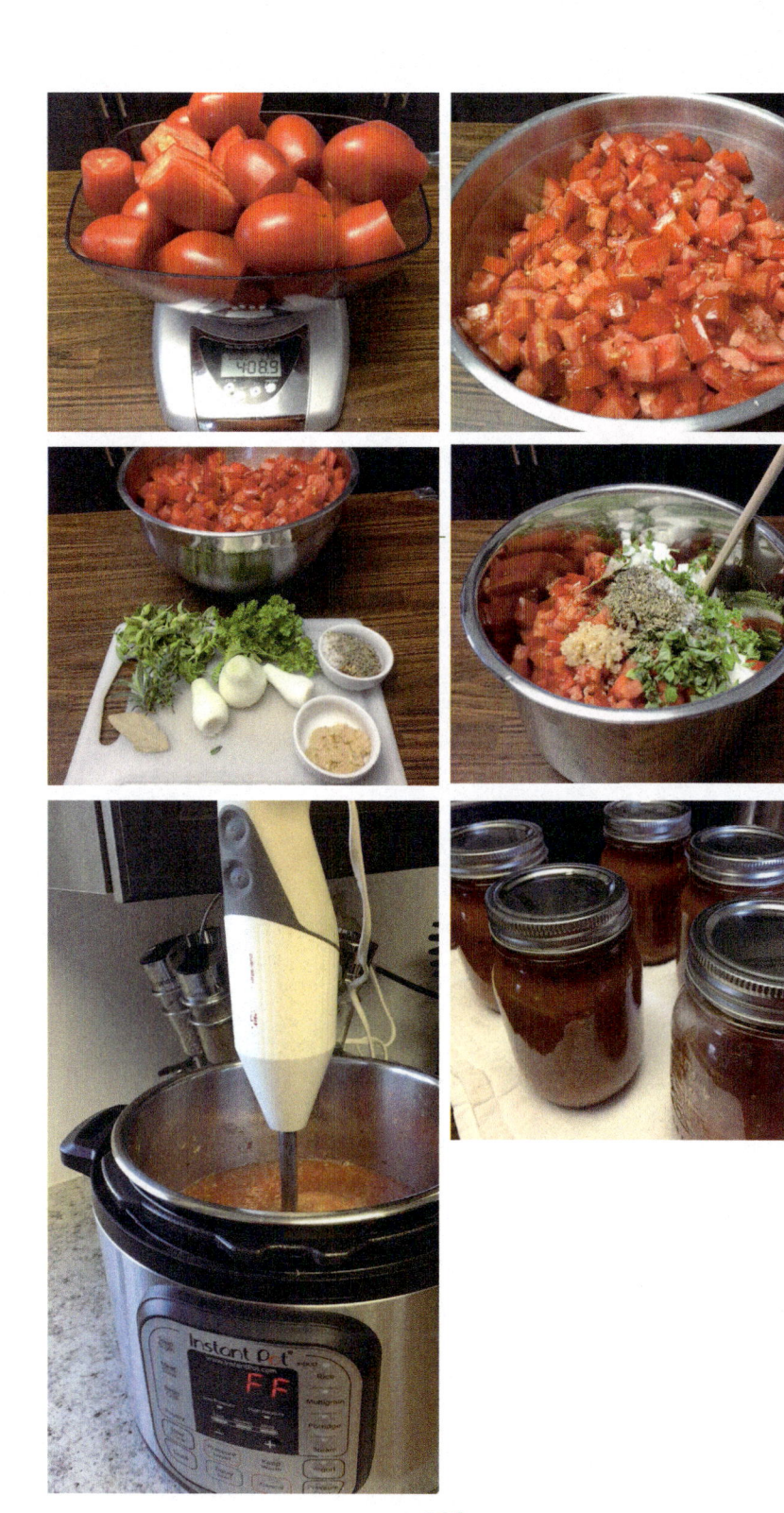

DESSERT RECIPES

Rice Pudding

| Vegan | Oil-free | | | Servings: 6 |

Rice pudding is always a nice dessert and the Instant Pot makes it super easy to make. Feel free to add some raisins and/or cinnamon and/or nutmeg.

INGREDIENTS

1 cup (225g) arborio rice*

4 cups (950 ml) cashew milk

½ cup (100g) sugar

1 teaspoon (5 ml) vanilla

¼ cup raisins (40g)(optional)

1 tablespoon cinnamon or nutmeg (15 ml) (optional)

This short grain rice produces a smoother pudding but regular white rice works, it is just a little grainier.

DIRECTIONS

1. Place all the ingredients in the inner liner of your Instant Pot and stir well.
2. Select the Porridge button and set the cooking time to 30 minutes.
3. When the cooking time is complete, allow a Full NPR (Natural Pressure Release) by allowing your Instant Pot to just sit (you can leave it on Keep Warm or just press the Cancel button) until the Float Valve drops on its own, indicating that all the pressure has been released.
4. Carefully remove the lid, stir well and serve or refrigerate for later use.

Nutritional Information per Serving:

Nutritional Information per Serving		
Servings	10	
Calories: 135		**Total fat:** 1.09g
Calories from fat: 9 (7%)		Saturated: 0.03g
Total Carbohydrates: 29.08g		Monounsaturated: 0.03g
Dietary Fiber: 0.96g		Polyunsaturated: 0.03g
Sugars: 12.83g		Trans fat: NA
Cholesterol: --	**Sodium:** 60mg	
Protein 1.70g	**Potassium** 16mg	
Vitamin A: --	**Vitamin C:** --	**Calcium:** --
Iron: 0.85mg	**Thiamin:** 0.11mg	**Niacin:** 0.82mg
Vitamin B6: 0.03mg	**Magnesium:** 4mg	**Folate:** 46µg

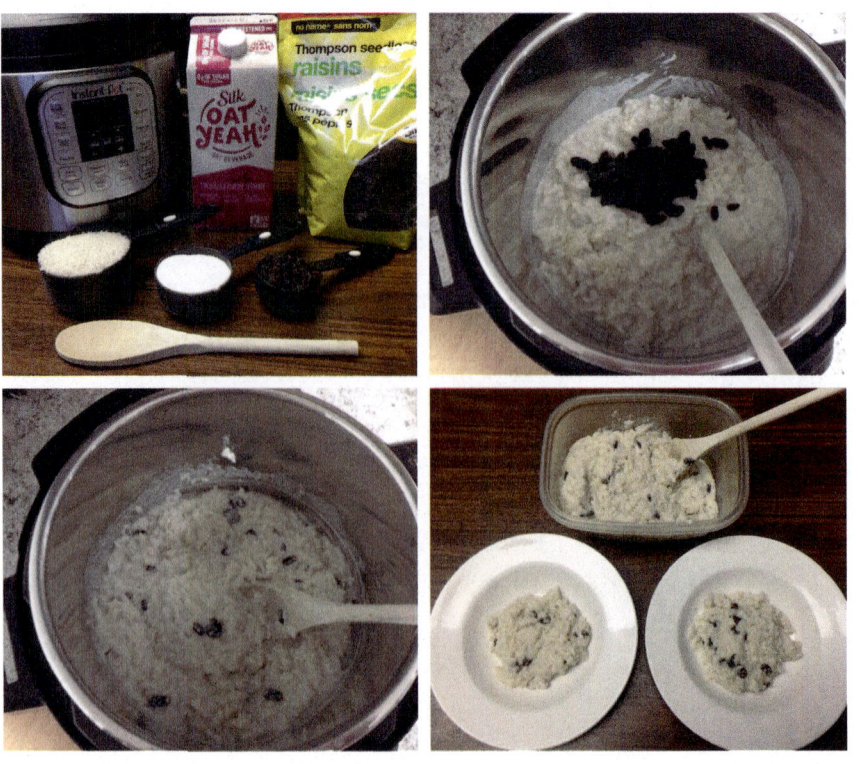

Easy Cheesecake for 2 (or 4)

Vegetarians Who Eat Eggs & Dairy	Servings 2/4

This is a quick and easy way to make great tasting cheesecake for 2 or 4 people. The "crust" is actually a whole, intact Digestive biscuit, eliminating the need to crush biscuits to make a crust.

INGREDIENTS FOR 2 (DOUBLE FOR 4)

2 Digestive biscuits

8 ounces (225g) cream cheese, at room temperature (use full fat - NOT the lite stuff)

¼ cup (50g) granulated sugar

1 large egg, at room temperature

1 tablespoon (15 ml) sour cream or Greek yogurt

1 teaspoon (5 ml) vanilla extract or almond flavoring

½ teaspoon (2.5 ml) grated lemon or orange rind (optional)

DIRECTIONS

1. Place one Digestive biscuit in each of 2 flat-bottomed, oven-safe ramekins. Set aside.
2. In a medium bowl, using an electric mixer on low, cream together the cream cheese and sugar.
3. Add the egg and mix well.
4. Add the sour cream and vanilla (or other flavoring) and mix well.
5. Divide the cream cheese mixture equally between the ramekins and smooth out the tops.
6. Add one cup (240 ml) of water to the inner pot of your Instant Pot and place the trivet in the inner pot as well.

7. Place the ramekins on top of the trivet.
8. Cover the ramekins with aluminum foil or silicone lids to prevent water from getting on the cheesecake as it cooks.
9. Close and lock the lid ensuring that the Pressure Valve is in the Sealing position.
10. Select the Pressure Cook/Manual button and set cooking time for 7 minutes.
11. Once cooking time is complete, allow a Natural Pressure Release for 10 minutes, then release the rest of the pressure by carefully turning the Pressure Valve from Sealing to Venting.
12. When all of the pressure has been released and the Float Valve has dropped, carefully remove the lid.
13. Press Cancel to turn the Instant Pot off.
14. Carefully remove the cheesecakes from the Instant Pot and allow them to cool on a wire rack until cool enough to handle (approximately 10 minutes).
15. Refrigerate the cheesecakes for at least one hour before serving.

Important Note:

Even if you double the recipe, DON'T double the cooking time. It stays the same whether you're making 2 or 4 individual cheesecakes.

Tip: If desired, you could spread about 1 to 1½ tablespoons (15 - 22.5 ml) of jam on top of each Digestive biscuit, before adding the cream cheese mixture to the ramekins. Then cook as above.

Nutritional Information per Serving:

Nutritional Information per Serving		
Servings 2		
Calories: 642	**Total fat:** 39.03g	
Calories from fat: 351 (54%)	Saturated: 24.14g	
Total Carbohydrates: 47.35g	Monounsaturated: 12.41g	
Dietary Fiber: 0.78g	Polyunsaturated: 2.48g	
Sugars: 37.77g	Trans fat: NA	
Cholesterol: 223mg	**Sodium:** 550mg	
Protein 11.37g	**Potassium** 257mg	
Vitamin A: 1695IU	**Vitamin C:** 0.70mg	**Calcium:** 140mg
Iron: 1.51mg	**Thiamin:** 0.11mg	**Niacin:** 0.66mg
Vitamin B6: 0.08mg	**Magnesium:** 13mg	**Folate:** 37µg

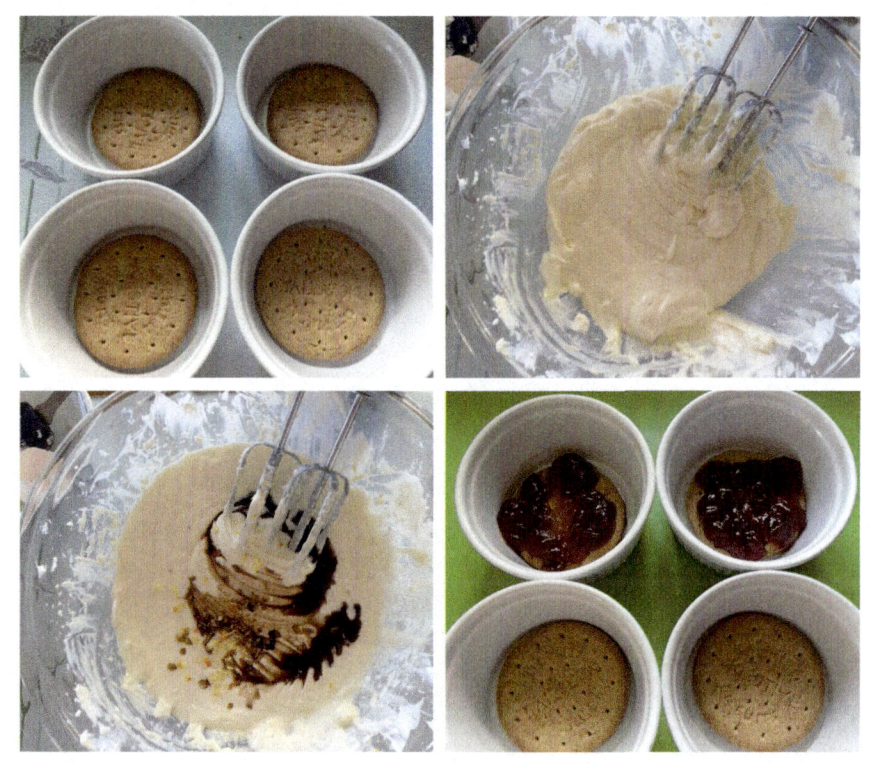

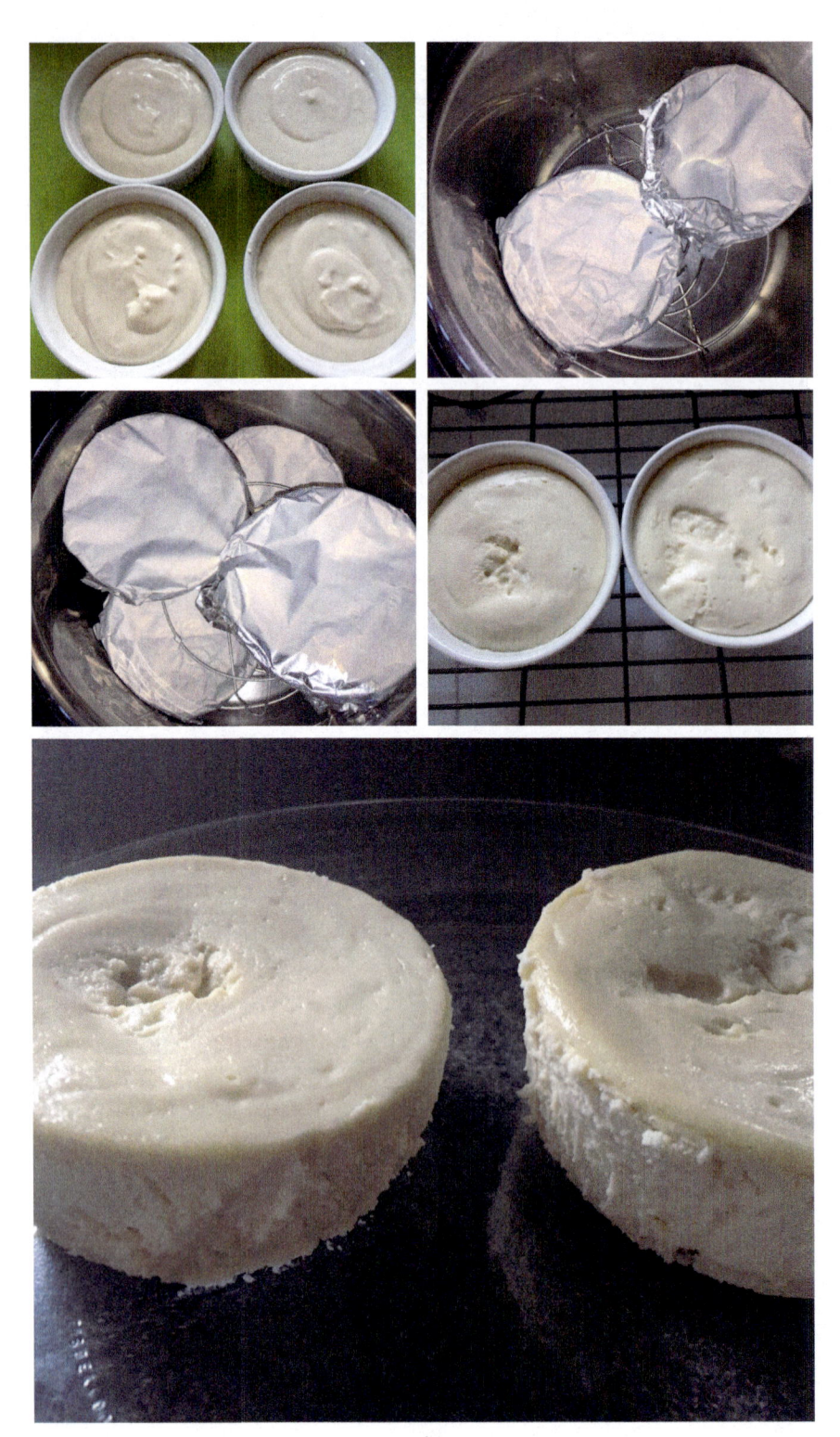

Lemon Curd

| Vegetarians Who Eat Eggs & Dairy | | Servings 32* |

*1 Tablespoon

*T*his recipe took a little trial and error before we got it just right. We also were able to use bitter oranges from our own orange trees in place of lemons and it came out great!

INGREDIENTS

4 large eggs

2 large egg yolks

1 cup (200g) granulated or caster sugar

1 cup (240 ml) lemon juice, freshly squeezed

1 pinch salt

1 tablespoon (5g) lemon zest

½ cup (120g) unsalted butter, room temperature

DIRECTIONS

1. In a 7" round x 3" deep (17cm round x 7.5 cm deep) oven-safe glass container, whisk together 4 large eggs and 2 large egg yolks.
2. Add 200g (1cup) granulated sugar and mix well.
3. Add a pinch of salt, 1 tbsp (5g) lemon zest, and 1 cup (240 ml) lemon juice. Mix until combined.
4. Wrap the glass container tightly with aluminum foil.
5. Pro Tip: be careful to avoid grating the bitter white pith when zesting the lemons.
6. Pour 1 cup (240 ml) cold water in the inner liner of your Instant Pot.

7. Place a trivet in the inner liner and carefully place the tightly wrapped glass container on the trivet.
8. Close and lock the lid ensuring the Pressure Valve is in the Sealing position.
9. Select the Pressure Cook/Manual button and set the cooking time for 10 minutes.
10. Once cooking time is complete, allow a 10-minute NPR (Natural Pressure Release).
11. In some cases, the Float Valve may drop after only 7-8 minutes, indicating that all the pressure has been released. However, DO NOT open the lid until the 10 minutes is up.
12. Carefully open the lid, remove the glass container and discard the aluminum foil.
13. At first, the mixture will look a lot like egg custard – don't panic!
14. Give the curd a few quick whisks with a silicone whisk and then add in, ¼ cup (60g) at a time, the room temperature unsalted butter, whisking after each addition to emulsify the butter with the egg mixture.
15. The lemon curd is now done and will thicken as it cools.
16. Pro Tip: You can filter out the lemon zest with a fine mesh strainer if you like. (We like to leave it in.)
17. Chill in the fridge for at least 4 hours before serving.

Nutritional Information per Serving:

Nutritional Information per Serving		
Servings 32		
Calories: 63	**Total fat:** 3.49g	
Calories from fat: 31 (49%)	Saturated: 2.12g	
Total Carbohydrates: 6.89g	Monounsaturated: 1.10g	
Dietary Fiber: 0.04g	Polyunsaturated: 0.27g	
Sugars: 6.47g	Trans fat: NA	
Cholesterol: 42mg	**Sodium:** 18mg	
Protein 1.01g	**Potassium** 18mg	
Vitamin A: 138IU	**Vitamin C:** 3.19mg	**Calcium:** 6mg
Iron: 0.15mg	**Thiamin:** 0.01mg	**Niacin:** 0.01mg
Vitamin B6: 0.02mg	**Magnesium:** 1mg	**Folate:** 6µg

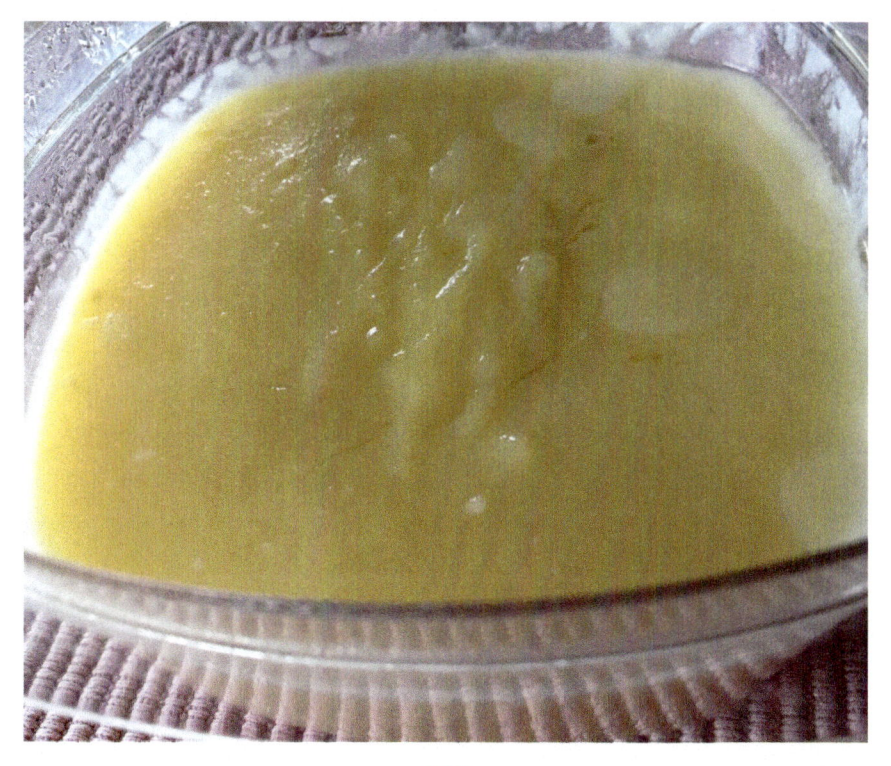

Cinnamon Apples Using the Pot-in-Pot Method

Vegan	Oil-free			Servings: 4

A quick and easy dessert that you can serve with Nice Cream (frozen bananas blended to ice cream consistency) – see our blog post for one variation of nice cream.

https://blog.reluctantvegetarians.com/hazelnut-coffee-nice-cream/

INGREDIENTS

4 medium Gala apples (or cooking apples of your choice), washed, cored and diced

¼ cup (45g) brown sugar

1 teaspoon (5 ml) vanilla

½ teaspoon (2.5 ml) cinnamon

DIRECTIONS

1. Combine all of the ingredients in an ovenproof bowl that will fit in the inner liner of your Instant Pot.
2. Place 1 cup (240 ml) of water in the inner liner of your Instant Pot and place the trivet in the inner liner as well.
3. Carefully place the bowl containing the apple mixture on the trivet.
4. Cover the bowl with a silicone lid or some aluminum foil to prevent water from getting into the bowl during cooking.
5. Close and lock the lid ensuring the Pressure Valve is in the Sealing position.
6. Select the Pressure Cook/Manual button and set the cooking time for 5 minutes.

7. Once cooking time is complete, allow a 5-minute NPR (Natural Pressure Release).
8. Then, release the rest of the pressure by carefully turning the Pressure Valve from Sealing to Venting.
9. When all of the pressure has been released and the Float Valve has dropped, carefully remove the lid.
10. Carefully remove the bowl to a heatproof surface and give the apple mixture a good stir.
11. Serve immediately or refrigerate for later use. This may freeze well, but we've never had any leftovers to give that a try.

Nutritional Information per Serving:

Nutritional Information per Serving		
Servings 4		
Calories: 154	**Total fat:** 0.00g	
Calories from fat: 0 (0%)	Saturated: 0.00g	
Total Carbohydrates: 37.41g	Monounsaturated: 0.00g	
Dietary Fiber: 4.13g	Polyunsaturated: 0.00g	
Sugars: 31.32g	Trans fat: NA	
Cholesterol: --	**Sodium:** 5mg	
Protein 0.46g	**Potassium** 206mg	
Vitamin A: 48IU	**Vitamin C:** 0.01mg	**Calcium:** 26mg
Iron: 0.33mg	**Thiamin:** 0.02mg	**Niacin:** 0.14mg
Vitamin B6: 0.07mg	**Magnesium:** 9mg	**Folate:** 5µg

148

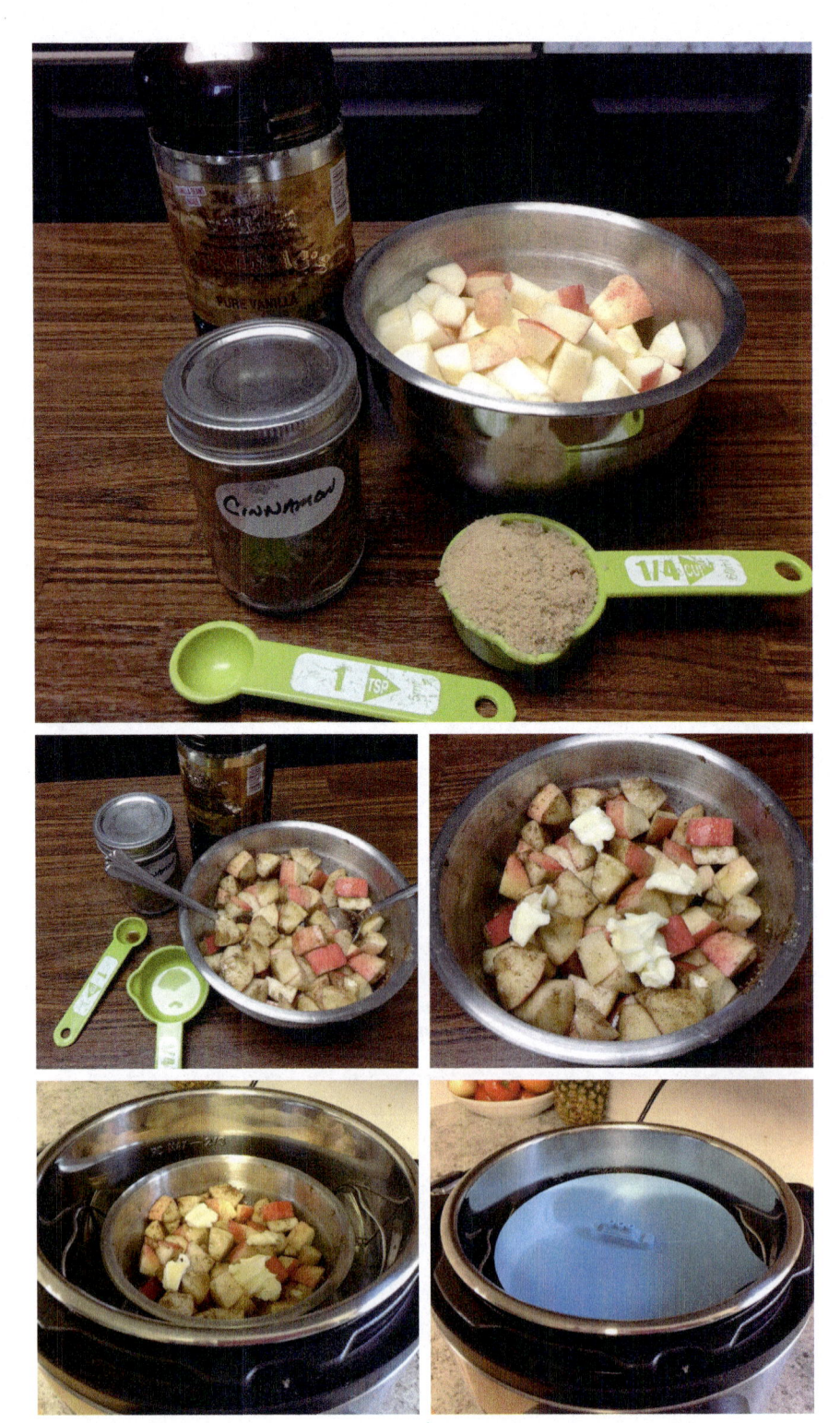

MISC RECIPES

Okay, this section is a "catch-all" for recipes that don't fit neatly into any other category. Just browse the recipes and you'll see what we mean.

Seasoned Diced Tomatoes

Vegan	Oil-free	WFPB		Servings: N/A

We have found, since we got our Instant Pot, that we are now more able to avoid canned items that we bought in abundance. We cook with diced tomatoes - a lot - and always had many, many tins in our pantry.

Now - we make our own diced tomatoes and can or freeze them for use in recipes.

This works well for us because we like to avoid all the added salt, etc. that you often find in canned foods. And, we know EXACTLY what's in our food.

INGREDIENTS

12 cups (2.4 Kg) fresh Roma tomatoes, diced

1½ teaspoons (7.5 ml) sea salt

1½ tablespoons (22.5 ml) dried basil

1 tablespoon (15 ml) dried thyme

1 tablespoon (15 ml) dried oregano

1½ teaspoons (7.5 ml) dried rosemary

6-8 cloves garlic, minced

½ cup (120 ml) tomato juice, optional depending on how juicy your tomatoes are

¼ cup (60 ml) lemon juice, preferably freshly squeezed but the bottled type will work, too

DIRECTIONS

1. Combine all of the ingredients in the inner pot of your Instant Pot and stir well.
2. Close and lock the lid ensuring the Pressure Valve is in the Sealing position.
3. Select Pressure Cook/Manual button and set the cooking time for 5 minutes.
4. When cooking time is complete do a Quick Release by carefully turning the Pressure Valve from Sealing to Venting.
5. Once all the pressure has been released and the Float Valve has dropped, carefully remove the lid.
6. Stir well.
7. Transfer the diced tomatoes to sterilized canning jars and allow to cool.
8. Refrigerate or freeze for later use.

   Note: If you decide to freeze your diced tomatoes, you may want to consider putting them in plastic containers or bags. We have experienced glass containers cracking in the freezer.

   Note: You can also can these diced tomatoes, if you prefer, using the water bath or steam method. How to can them is beyond the scope of this book. For more information on safe home canning, you may want to visit the National Center for Home Food Preservation at: https://nchfp.uga.edu/publications/publications_usda.html

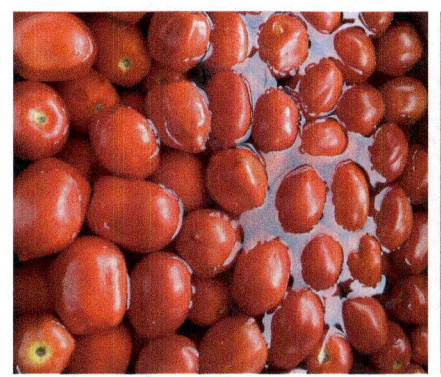

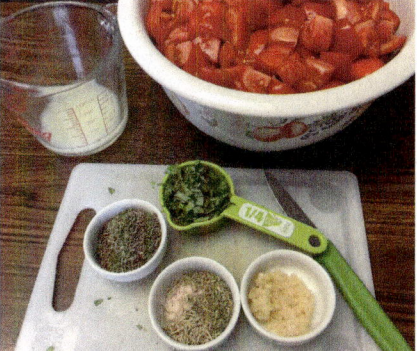

Nutritional Information per Serving:

Nutritional Information per Serving		
Servings 18		
Calories: 26	**Total fat:** 0.20g	
Calories from fat: 1 (6%)	Saturated: 0.04g	
Total Carbohydrates: 5.95g	Monounsaturated: 0.04g	
Dietary Fiber: 1.73g	Polyunsaturated: 0.11g	
Sugars: 3.44g	Trans fat: NA	
Cholesterol: --	**Sodium:** 200mg	
Protein 1.26g	**Potassium** 314mg	
Vitamin A: 1055IU	**Vitamin C:** 23.08mg	**Calcium:** 24mg
Iron: 0.71mg	**Thiamin:** 0.05mg	**Niacin:** 0.79mg
Vitamin B6: 0.12mg	**Magnesium:** 15mg	**Folate:** 21µg

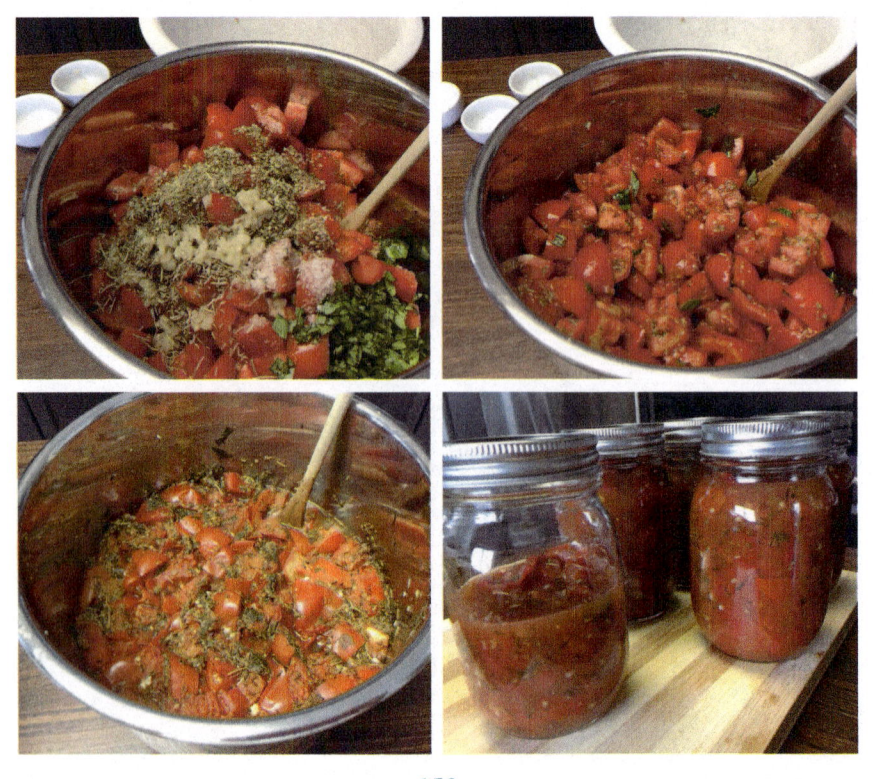

Corn Salsa

| Vegan | Oil-free | WFPB | | Servings: 30 |

*½ cup servings

*T*his is another recipe that doesn't last long in our house. It makes a great snack with some homemade (or store bought) tortilla chips and some refried beans (recipe below).

INGREDIENTS

12 cups (2.4 Kg) Roma (plum) tomatoes, diced

2 stalks celery, diced

1 medium bell pepper, diced, red or green

3 large yellow onions, diced

½ cup (52g) jalapeño, diced

½ cup (120 ml) tomato paste

½ cup (120 ml) spaghetti sauce, your choice or crushed tomatoes

½ cup (120 ml) white vinegar

3 tablespoons (45 ml) sugar

1 tablespoon (15 ml) sea salt

6 cloves garlic, minced

1 teaspoon (5 ml) cayenne pepper

2 cups (350g) corn, fresh or frozen

DIRECTIONS

1. Combine all of the ingredients in the inner pot of your Instant Pot and stir well.
2. Close and lock the lid ensuring the Pressure Valve is in the Sealing position.

3. Select the Pressure Cook/Manual button and set the cooking time for 5 minutes.
4. When cooking time is complete do a 10-minute Natural Pressure Release followed by a Quick Release by carefully turning the Pressure valve from Sealing to Venting.
5. Once all the pressure has been released and the Float Valve has dropped, carefully remove the lid.
6. Stir well.
7. Transfer the salsa to sterilized canning jars and allow to cool.
8. Refrigerate or freeze for later use.
9. Note: If you decide to freeze your salsa, you may want to consider using plastic containers or bags. We have experienced glass containers cracking in the freezer.
10. Note: You can also can this salsa, if you prefer, using the water bath or steam method. How to can them is beyond the scope of this book. For more information on safe home canning, you may want to visit the National Center for Home Food Preservation at: https://nchfp.uga.edu/publications/publications_usda.html

Nutritional Information per Serving:

Nutritional Information per Serving	
Servings 30	
Calories: 39	**Total fat:** 0.26g
Calories from fat: 2 (5%)	Saturated: 0.05g
Total Carbohydrates: 8.87g	Monounsaturated: 0.07g
Dietary Fiber: 1.80g	Polyunsaturated: 0.14g
Sugars: 4.74g	Trans fat: NA
Cholesterol: --	**Sodium:** 263mg
Protein 1.47g	**Potassium** 302mg
Vitamin A: 787IU	**Vitamin C:** 19.23mg	**Calcium:** 16mg
Iron: 0.59mg	**Thiamin:** 0.06mg	**Niacin:** 0.87mg
Vitamin B6: 0.12mg	**Magnesium:** 16mg	**Folate:** 21µg

155

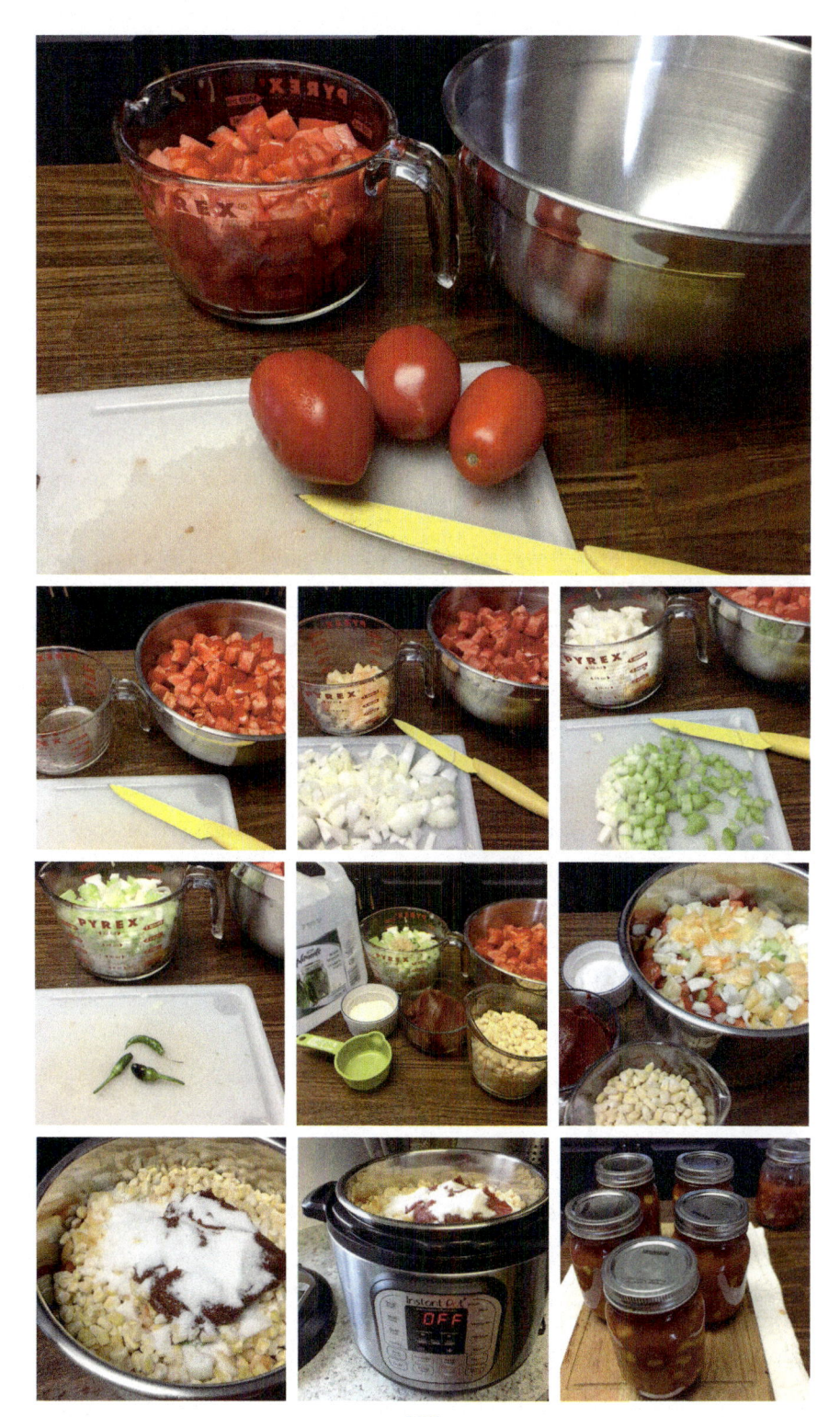

Easy Refried Beans

Vegan	WFPB	Servings: 2

We thought refried beans would be difficult to make. We love refried beans, however, they're usually pretty expensive to buy in cans. Solution? Make them in the Instant Pot.

We were amazed at how easy and inexpensive it is to make this Mexican staple. We will never buy another can of refried beans again!

So, don't be intimidated. This recipe is really easy and I'm sure you'll get rave reviews.

INGREDIENTS

26 ounces (750g) dried pinto beans (or substitute Romano beans if you can't find pinto beans)

1½ cups (225g) onion, chopped

4-5 garlic cloves, roughly chopped

1 jalapeño pepper, seeded and chopped

1 tablespoon (15 ml) dried oregano

2 teaspoons (10 ml) ground cumin

½ teaspoon (2.5 ml) ground black pepper

3 tablespoons (35g) coconut oil

4 cups (950 ml) vegetable broth

2 cups (475 ml) water

1-2 teaspoons (5-10 ml) sea salt (added after cooking is complete)

DIRECTIONS

1. In a large bowl, soak the dried beans in enough water to cover, for approximately 15 minutes.
2. Add all of the other ingredients (except the salt) to the inner liner of your Instant Pot.
3. Drain the beans you set aside to soak and rinse.
4. Add the beans to the rest of the ingredients and stir.
5. Close and lock the lid, ensuring the Pressure Valve is in the Sealing position.
6. Select the Bean/Chili button and set cooking time to 45 minutes.
7. Once cooking time is complete, allow a full Natural Pressure Release (this can take some time - we waited for almost 50 minutes). A complete Natural Pressure Release means that you wait until the pin drops on its own without switching the Pressure Valve to Venting.
8. Once the pressure has released on its own and the Float Valve has dropped, open the lid, remove the inner liner carefully (it's going to be really hot) and place it on a heat-proof surface.
9. Add the sea salt, to taste.
10. Use an immersion blender to achieve the desired consistency.

Nutritional Information per Serving:

Nutritional Information per Serving	
Servings	24
Calories: 140	**Total fat:** 1.92g
Calories from fat: 17 (12%)	Saturated: 1.56g
Total Carbohydrates: 23.64g	Monounsaturated: 0.20g
Dietary Fiber: 5.54g	Polyunsaturated: 0.17g
Sugars: 2.58g	Trans fat: NA
Cholesterol: --	**Sodium:** 291mg
Protein 7.08g	**Potassium** 491mg
Vitamin A: 96IU	**Vitamin C:** 5.55mg	**Calcium:** 50mg
Iron: 1.85mg	**Thiamin:** 0.24mg	**Niacin:** 0.43mg
Vitamin B6: 0.20mg	**Magnesium:** 59mg	**Folate:** 168µg

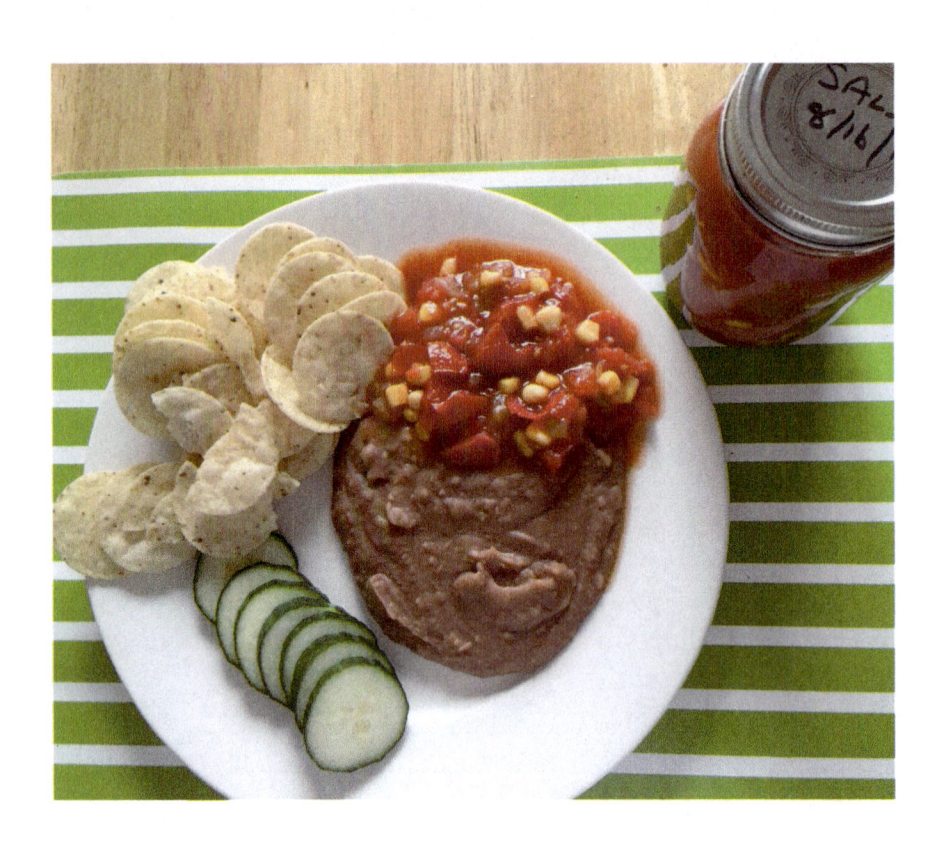

No Soak Beans

| Vegan | Oil-free | WFPB | | |

To use immediately or to freeze for future use

We don't buy canned beans anymore. We cook our own in our Instant Pot and freeze them in 1½ to 2 cup packages (just the right size for the recipes we like).

Here's how you can make your own. See the instructions for different beans below.

INGREDIENTS

16 ounces (454g) dry beans

5 cups (1.2 L) vegetable broth or water (or a combination of both)

2 - 3 garlic cloves, roughly chopped (optional)

½ yellow onion, roughly chopped (optional)

1-2 Bay leaves (optional)

DIRECTIONS

1. For all of the beans, be sure to rinse them well first and discard any broken beans or stones (yes, you might actually find some stones in your dried beans).

BLACK BEANS

1. Place all of the ingredients in your Instant Pot and stir.
2. Note: with black beans you may want to add 1 teaspoon (5 ml) of cumin (optional).

3. Close the lid of your Instant Pot and ensure that the Pressure Valve is in the Sealing position.
4. Select Bean/Chili button and set the cooking time for 22 minutes.
5. When cooking time is complete, allow a full Natural Pressure Release (can take up to 30 minutes or more).
6. Once the pressure has released fully, carefully remove the lid and give the beans a good stir.

CHICKPEAS (GARBANZO BEANS)

1. Place all of the ingredients in your Instant Pot and stir.
2. Close the lid of your Instant Pot and ensure that the Pressure Valve is in the Sealing position.
3. Select Bean/Chili button and set cooking time for 35 minutes.
4. When cooking time is complete, allow a full Natural Pressure Release (can take up to 30 minutes or more).
5. Once the pressure has released fully, carefully remove the lid and give the beans a good stir.
6. Note: Be sure to save the leftover water from chickpeas. It's called aquafaba and you'll find lots of recipes that use it.

WHITE BEANS (NAVY BEANS, GREAT NORTHERN BEANS, ETC.)

1. Place all of the ingredients in your Instant Pot and stir.
2. Close the lid of your Instant Pot and ensure that the valve is in the Sealing position.
3. Select Bean/Chili mode and set cooking time for 20 minutes if the beans are small, 25 minutes if they are larger.
4. When cooking time is complete, allow a full Natural Pressure Release (can take up to 30 minutes or more).
5. Once the pressure has released fully, carefully remove the lid and give the beans a good stir.

KIDNEY BEANS

1. Kidney beans are an exception to the "no soak" method. You should soak kidney beans, in fresh water, for at least a couple of hours.

Then drain and rinse before continuing with the cooking method below:

2. Place all of the ingredients in your Instant Pot and stir.
3. Close the lid of your Instant Pot and ensure that the Pressure Valve is in the Sealing position.
4. Select Bean/Chili button and set cooking time for 25 minutes.
5. When cooking time is complete, allow a full Natural Pressure Release (can take up to 30 minutes or more).
6. Once the pressure has released fully, carefully remove the lid and give the beans a good stir.

FOR ALL COOKED BEANS

Allow the beans to cool and then package approximately 1½ - 2 cups in a freezer bag.

Try to get most of the air out of the bag and seal.

Hint: Lay the bags as flat as you can (being very careful not to let the contents leak out, and gently, oh so gently, get out as much air as you can) and freeze them flat.

This way, they not only freeze faster, they'll also thaw faster when you want to use them.

Note: Don't forget to label each bag with what they are and the date you packaged and froze them.

Nutritional Information per Serving:

All beans are a nutritious addition to any diet

The exact quantity of nutrients and mix of micro nutrients will, of course, depend on the type of bean you choose.

Homemade Vegetable Broth

Vegan	Oil-free	WFPB	

It's amazingly easy to make your own vegetable broth in an Instant Pot and it's virtually cost-free.

You probably throw away a fair bit of vegetable matter. The thick stalks of broccoli, outside cabbage leaves, potato and carrot peelings, etc. Instead of throwing it all in the garbage, put it in a plastic bag in your freezer. When you have collected a bag full you can make some Instant Pot Broth.

This is a lot healthier than buying commercial broth and you know exactly what goes into it.

HERE'S THE TYPE OF VEGETABLE PEELINGS AND BITS YOU SHOULD SAVE:

- carrot peelings and ends
- celery leaves and ends
- tomato cores and ends
- potato peelings
- yam (sweet potato) peelings
- outer bits of onions (not the yellow part, but the tough outer white layer)
- garlic (the end you cut off before mincing, not the papery stuff)
- apple cores
- lettuce leaves that have wilted (iceberg, romaine, etc.)
- summer squash and zucchini ends
- mushroom stems
- pea pods

- beet greens
- cucumber ends

ADD THE FOLLOWING SPARINGLY BECAUSE OF THEIR SOMEWHAT OVERWHELMING FLAVOR AND ODOR

- cabbage leaves
- broccoli stems
- cauliflower cores
- kale stems

We use a one-gallon Ziploc™ Freezer Bag (approximately 10" x 10" or 25 cm x 25 cm) to collect the peelings, etc. and make broth once the bag is full.

INGREDIENTS

1 bag of saved frozen vegetable peelings and bits

12 cups (2.8L) water, approximately

1-2 bay leaves, optional

DIRECTIONS

1. Place the water and the contents of your saved bag of vegetable scraps in your Instant Pot's inner pot.
2. Close and lock the lid ensuring the pressure valve is in the Sealing position.
3. Select the Soup/Broth button and set the cooking time for 2 hours (120 minutes).
4. Once cooking time is complete, allow a complete Natural Pressure Release. That means just turning the Instant Pot off and waiting for the Float Valve to drop on its own (This can take an hour or more).
5. Once the pressure has completely released, carefully open and remove the lid.
6. Carefully, using oven mitts, remove the inner pot to a heatproof surface and allow to cool.
7. Use a slotted spoon to remove all the large pieces of the vegetables. (Tip: You can put this in your compost or blend it with some water and feed it to your plants. They love it!)

8. Then strain the rest of the liquid through a fine sieve and discard any additional vegetable matter (as mentioned above).

   Place the vegetable broth in containers and freeze for later use. (Tip: Measure the amount of broth you put in each container and label the container with the amount. You can put frozen vegetable broth directly into an Instant Pot recipe.)

Here's a link to a short video we made on how to make vegetable broth in your Instant Pot -

https://reluctantvegetarians.com/how-to-make-vegetable-broth-in-an-instant-pot/

Nutritional Information per Serving:

The additional flavor and nutrition provided by the varied contents of the broth is small but it is more than just plain water.

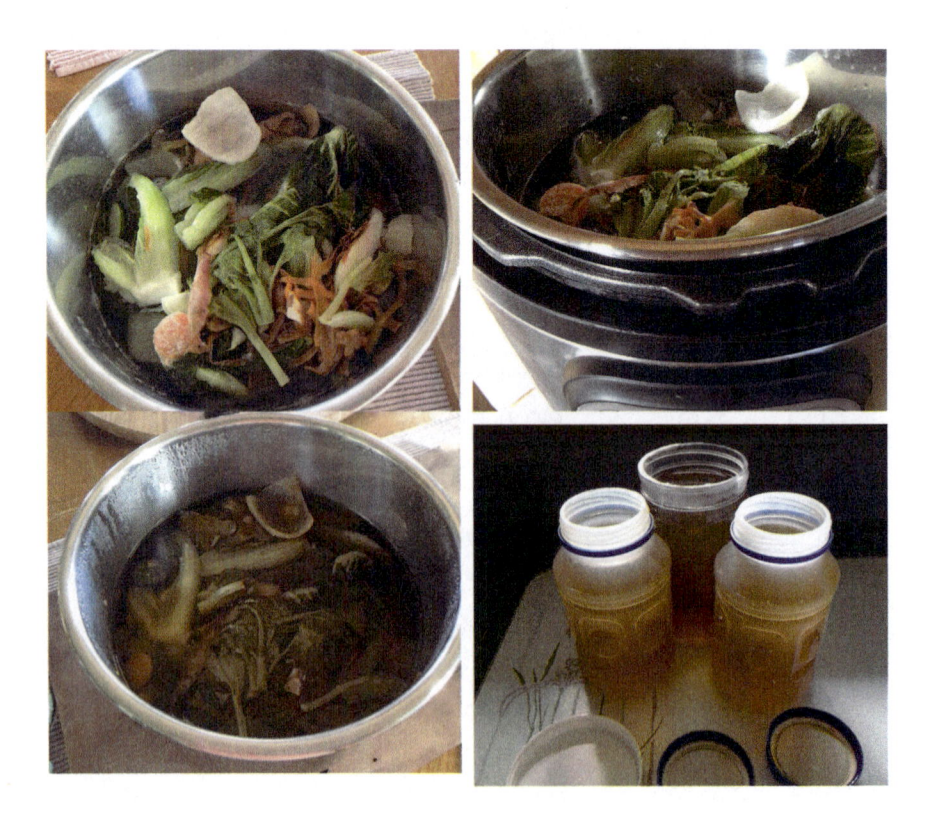

BONUS SECTION

We write a lot of books and we hope you will always be happy with your purchases from us.

"Under promise and over deliver," has always been a motto of ours, so to thank you for your purchase we would like to give you a free bonus.

Just go to -

https://fun.reluctantvegetarians.com/veganbonus

to claim it.

Just One More Thing

- Did you enjoy reading this book?
- Do you think you got good value?
- Did it deliver what we promised in the description?

If you answered no to any of the questions above please return this book for a full refund. If you answered yes, please leave a review so that others will feel confident buying their own copy of this book.

Reviews are incredibly important to independent authors so we sincerely hope you will do us the courtesy of leaving a review for your fellow Reluctant Vegetarians.

We know you are busy and it will take a little bit of your time to leave the review so it's only fair we offer a small gift in return. The truth is you can get the gift if you leave a review or not, but we hope you do.

Just go to the URL below to claim it.

Thank you,

Geoff and Vicky Wells

Your reward is waiting for you at:

https://fun.reluctantvegetarians.com/veganreward

Other Books In The Reluctant Vegetarian Series

This is the sixth book in the Reluctant Vegetarian series. The other five are available from Amazon in print, ebook, large print and audio editions.

Many of our books have been translated into Spanish, French Italian, Portuguese, Afrikaans and Japanese.

Check out any of these books by going to:

https://geezerguides.com or use the Amazon links below each book in the following pages

OUR OTHER WEBSITES YOU MIGHT ENJOY

https://reluctantvegetarians.com

https://blog.reluctantvegetarians.com

https://wfpbunderpressure.com

https://instantpotvideorecipes.com

Our Facebook Pages:

https://www.facebook.com/ReluctantVegetarians/

https://www.facebook.com/InstantPotVideoRecipes/

https://www.facebook.com/WFPBunderpressure

A Guide to Juicing, Raw Foods & Superfoods

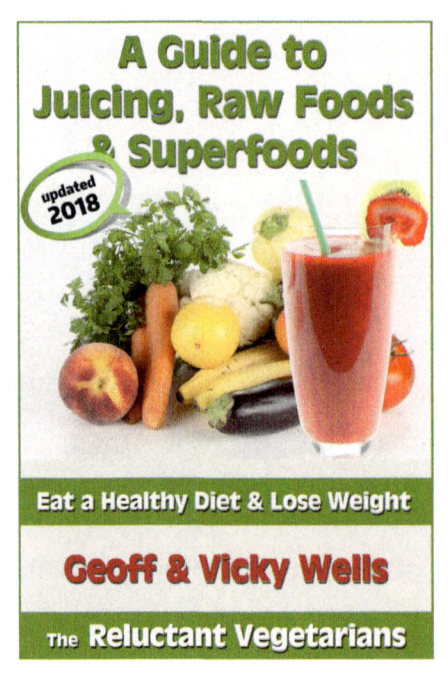

A Guide to Juicing, Raw Foods & Superfoods is a compendium of information that not only highlights the amazing benefits of adding juicing, raw foods and Superfoods to your diet, it also includes over 30 delicious and easy to follow recipes.

It is the first step on your journey to finding the best options for a healthy lifestyle.

The authors, Geoff and Vicky Wells, have already begun this journey and are seeing some remarkable results. They are aware that there is an ever-increasing group of people who are looking for natural solutions to their health problems and have sought to provide a number of solutions from their own experiences.

The items that are recommended can easily be found in any local farmers market or grocery store and, if your shopping is properly planned, it will not put a strain on your grocery budget.

Both the information and tasty recipes in this book are a must-have for any individual who wants to achieve optimal health. It also serves as a reference for those who are just beginning to research the benefits of a juicing, raw foods and Superfoods diet.

Now is always the best time to begin your journey to a fitter, longer, healthier life.

Please note that this book is NOT about centrifugal juicing but rather about using a powerful blender to reduce fruits and vegetables to a juice without removing any fiber.

Here Are Just A Few Headings From Our Linked Table of Contents

What Is Juicing?

What Is A Raw Food Diet?

What Are Superfoods?

What Are the Benefits of Juicing?

What Are the Benefits of Eating Raw Foods and Superfoods?

More Than 30 Recipes:

- Almond Milk
- Cashew Milk
- Chocolate and Coconut Smoothie
- Fresh From The Garden Vegetable Cocktail
- Geoff's Famous Hummus
- Goodness Gracious Green
- Hot Veggie Drink
- Minty Green Refresher
- Multi-Bean Salad
- Peachy Green Smoothie
- Peppered Strawberries
- Raw Fruit Salad
- Raw Veggies and Dip
- Rice Milk
- Tomato, Cucumber and Cilantro Salad
- Very Berry Smoothie
- Vicky's Granola
- Almost Waldorf Salad (No Mayo)
- Nut Butter
- Plus Many More

Available from Amazon in Print and eBook editions

https://amzn.to/3fMb4xg

Super 3 Day Detox Soup & Smoothie Plan

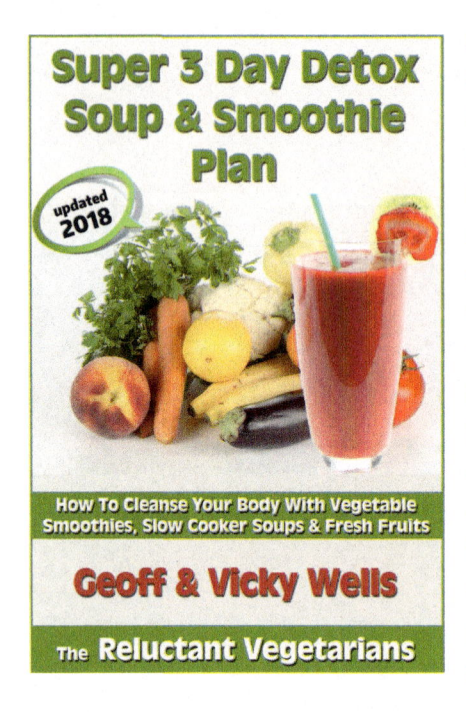

Super 3 Day Detox Soup & Smoothie Plan is an easy to follow three-day detox plan that consists of delicious smoothies for breakfast and lunch, a hot and tasty slow cooker soup/stew for dinner, and fresh mixed fruit for dessert.

This plan fits a busy lifestyle, too, because you can pre-make your lunch smoothies and take them with you. You can also set up your slow cooker in the morning and have dinner all ready for you when you get home.

Here's some insight into what's included in this book:

A Candid Interview With the Authors

What Are the Benefits of a Detox Program?

What Are The Potential Side Effects of a Detox Program?

Tips for Choosing Your Fruits, Vegetables and Herbs
- Why Organic is Best
- Why Raw is Best

The Foods We Used and Why
- From Apples to Turmeric

What the Colors of Foods Mean
- Red, Orange, Yellow, Green, Blue, Purple and White

Most and Least Contaminated Fruits and Vegetables
- 12 Most Contaminated Foods
- 12 Least Contaminated Foods

What NOT to Consume While Detoxing

Staying Hydrated While Detoxing

Commitment

Mindset

Preparation

Food Safety

The 3-Day Detox Program
- The 3-Day Plan
- Detox Recipes
- The Detox Recipes for Breakfast, Lunch, Dinner and Dessert
- Vitamin Detox Water
- Bonus Recipe
- Homemade Vegetable Wash

Get this book now and get started on your 3-day detox program!

https://amzn.to/37l1cqB

Our Favorite Detox & Weight Loss Slow Cooker Recipes

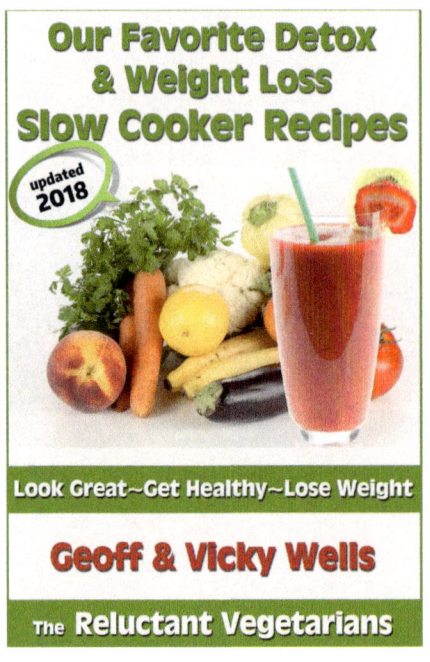

We love slow cooker meals because they are easy, convenient and tasty. Even better are slow cooker meals that help you lose weight and get healthy.

You'll find that when you eat a vegetarian or vegan diet, you'll be eating a lot more nutrient-dense food while keeping your calories very low.

That's not to say that ALL vegan and vegetarian food is low calorie. You'll still need to watch your intake of fats and higher calorie foods, but you'll also find that you retain the "full" feeling longer because your body is getting more of the nutrients it needs.

Some of the recipes are good for detox and they are noted as such. All of the recipes are vegetarian or vegan and most of them will help you to lose weight as well.

Here's the recipes you'll find. And yes, you make them in your slow cooker:

Breakfast

- Apple Cinnamon Oatmeal
- Bread Pudding for Breakfast
- Fruit & Nut Breakfast Oatmeal
- Multi-Grain Hot Cereal
- Pear and Chai Breakfast Cake
- Spicy Breakfast Risotto

Lunch and Dinner

- Autumn Harvest Stew
- Baby Spinach with White Beans

- Basic Vegetarian/Vegan Baked Beans
- Black Bean Stew
- Broccoli and Cauliflower
- Detox Soup
- Butternut Squash and Parsnip Soup
- Cabbage and Apple Soup
- Cabbage and Apple Side Dish
- Canadian Maple Baked Beans
- Chunky Root Vegetable Stew
- Coconut Curry Stew
- Easy Pinto Beans
- Hearty Barley and Lentil Stew
- Italian Style Beans with Sun Dried Tomatoes and Black Olives
- Lentil Chili
- Mexican Chickpeas
- Mushroom and Spinach Quiche
- Red Cabbage and Carrot Detox Soup
- Sicilian-Style Fava Beans
- Spaghetti Sauce
- Split Pea and Cabbage Stew
- Tomato and Kale Detox Soup
- Vegetable and Lentil Stew

Dessert

- Chocolate Peanut Butter Cake
- Cranberry Peach Cobbler
- Fruity Cobbler
- Pumpkin Nut Bread
- Rice Pudding
- Bonus Recipe - Homemade Pumpkin Pie Spice

Some of the dessert recipes are a little higher in calories so use them sparingly.

https://amzn.to/37hCDdV

Reluctant Vegetarians 3-Book Box Set

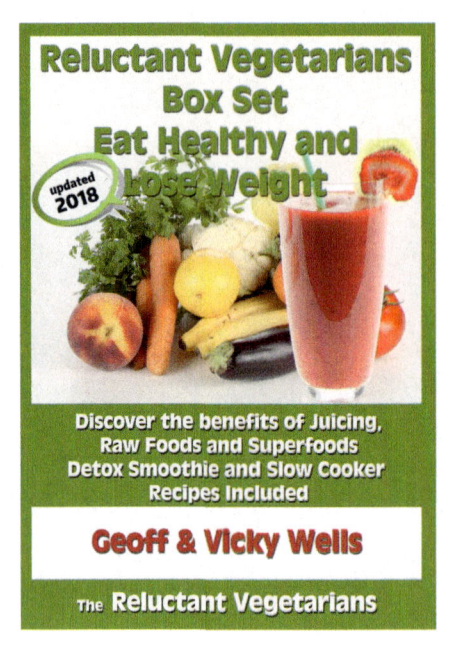

Three great books in one!

This set includes:

Volume 1:

A Guide to Juicing, Raw Foods and Super Foods: Eat a Healthy Diet and Lose Weight which covers:

- the benefits of juicing
- the benefits of raw foods
- the benefits of superfoods
- combining all the benefits for a healthy lifestyle
- Lots of Recipes:
- how to make non-dairy milk - almond, cashew, rice coconut
- 18 juices, smoothies and drinks recipes
- 8 raw food salad recipes

Additional Recipes for:

- granola
- nut butter
- peppered strawberries
- raw apple sauce
- hummus
- and more …

Volume 2:

Super 3-Day Detox Soup & Smoothie Plan: How to Cleanse YourBody with Vegetable Smoothies, Slow Cooker Soups & FreshFruits which covers:

- the benefits of a detox program
- 3-day menu plan
- recipes for breakfast, lunch, dinner and desserts for ALL three days

Bonus vitamin detox water recipe

Volume 3:

Our Favorite Detox & Weight Lose Slow Cooker Recipes: Look Great - Get Healthy - Lose Weight which covers:

- vegetarian vs vegan - what's the difference?
- why buy organic
- avoiding GMOs
- freezing fresh fruit
- 8 amazing breakfast recipes
- over 25 easy lunch/dinner recipes
- 5 tasty dessert recipes

Bonus make your own pumpkin spice recipe

Start your journey to a healthier lifestyle today with this amazing box set from the Reluctant Vegetarians.

Learn about juicing, raw foods, super foods, healthy eating, good-for-you recipes and more …

Explore which foods to choose, and why, to begin and to maintain a healthy lifestyle.

Detox with any easy to follow 3-day plan.

Discover all kinds of recipes that incorporate healthy, nutritious foods while being easy to prepare and tasty, too.

https://amzn.to/3q9HDtJ

How Do Vegans Get Their Protein?

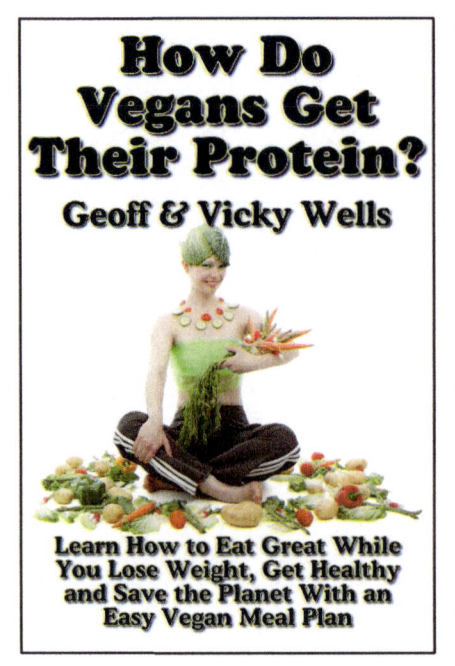

New for 2020!

This new book from Geoff and Vicky Wells explains how Vegans (and vegetarians, too) get their protein. It addresses the major concerns of most non-vegans/vegetarians about how they can include sufficient protein in their diet without resorting to animal products.

This information-packed book is written in three sections:

Part I

Chapter 1 - What is a Vegan Diet

Chapter 2 - Important Food Groups for a Healthy Vegan Diet

Chapter 3 - Overview of a Protein-Rich Vegan Diet

Chapter 4 - Best Vegan Foods for Weight Management & Muscle Building

Chapter 5 - Vegan Diet and Exercise

Chapter 6 - Mistakes to Avoid on a Vegan Diet

Part II

This section provides an entire week's worth of suggested, protein-rich, vegan meals for breakfast, lunch, dinner, desserts and snacks.

Part III

This section contains over 50 high-protein vegan recipes for breakfast, lunch, dinner, desserts and snacks.

Here's just a sampling of some of the recipes:

Breakfast

- Vicky's Favorite Granola
- Breakfast "Sausage" Patties
- Gluten-Free, Sugar-Free Vegan Pancakes

- Several Smoothie Recipes

and more …

Lunch

- Chickpea "No-Egg" Salad
- Basic Baked Beans
- Mexican Style Bean Salad
- Vegan Carrot Hot Dogs

and more …

Dinner

- Roasted Cauliflower Dinner (complete with gravy!)
- Geoff's Favorite "No-Meat" Loaf
- Chickpea Pot Pie
- Vegan Roasted Vegetable Medley

and more …

Soups

- Carrot & Pumpkin Soup
- Split Pea, Apple and Cabbage Soup
- Corn and Cabbage Chowder
- and more …

Condiments & Sauces

- Geoff's Famous Hummus
- Spaghetti Sauce
- Salad Dressings
- Sugar-Free Stir Fry Sauce

and more …

Desserts

- Piña Colada Nice Cream
- Banana Cake
- Strawberry Muffins
- Tropical Dream Smoothie

Get your copy today to get healthy, lose weight and save the planet!

https://amzn.to/37iSxVo

Printed in Great Britain
by Amazon